BodySkills

A MOTOR DEVELOPMENT CURRICULUM FOR CHILDREN

Manual

JUDY K. WERDER
ROBERT H. BRUININKS

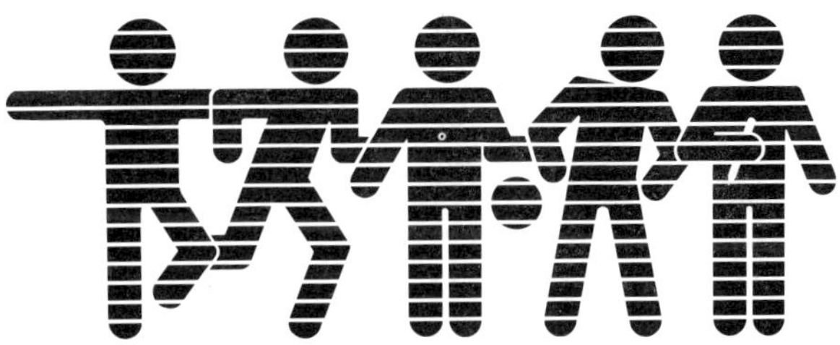

AGS®
American Guidance Service
Circle Pines, Minnesota 55014-1796

AGS staff participating in the development and production of this publication

Project Team

Karen Dahlen, Project Editor
Mary Kaye Kuzma, Production Coordinator
Lynn Estuesta, Marketing Associate

Dorothy Chapman, Director of Program Development
Lois Welshons, Art Editor
Lynne Cromwell, Production Manager
Maureen Wilson, Art Director
Elizabeth Berry, Sylvia Carsen, Production Artists

Design

Terry Dugan, Terry Dugan Design

Illustrations

Vergal Buescher, Buescher and Associates

Printed in the United States of America

Library of Congress Catalog Card Number: 87-072688

ISBN: 0-88671-185-1

A 10 9 8 7 6 5 4 3 2 1

Contents

Illustrations 5
Acknowledgments 7
Chapter 1 Introduction 9
Features 9
Organization 11
Materials 11
Scope and Structure of the *Body Skills* Curriculum 12
Body Skills Assessment System 14
Applications 15

Chapter 2 Using the *Body Skills* Curriculum 17
Skill Folders and Activity Cards 17
Skill Folders 17
Activity Cards 18
Teaching the Activities 22
Monitoring Progress While Teaching 23
Developing Lesson Plans 26
Planning an Assessment Schedule 29

Chapter 3 Assessment, Instructional Planning, and Evaluation 31
Assessment Strategies 31
Instructions for the MSI 36
Interpreting Assessment Results for Instructional Planning 37
Developing Group and Individual Educational Plans 43
A Case Study 46
Evaluation 50
Student Evaluation 50
Program Evaluation 55

Chapter 4 Research and Development 59
Rationale 59
Procedural Model for Curriculum Development 60
Program Structure and Content 61
Program Goals and Objectives 62
Designing the Curriculum 63
Development of Prototype Materials 66

Chapter 5 Test Information and Equating Study 71
Technical Characteristics of the *Bruininks-Oseretsky Test* 71
Equating *Bruininks-Oseretsky Test* and MSI Score Levels 72
Technical Characteristics of the MSI 74

Appendixes
Appendix A Directions for Administering and Scoring the Motor Skills Inventory 77
Appendix B Adaptations for Students with Handicapping Conditions 110
Appendix C *Body Skills* Materials 126
Appendix D Sample Yearly Program Plan Using the *Body Skills* Curriculum 130
Appendix E Field Testers 135
Glossary 139
References 141

Illustrations

Figures

Figure 1.1	Overview of the *Body Skills* curriculum	10
Figure 1.2	Organization and content of the Motor Skills Inventory (MSI)	14
Figure 1.3	Relationship between subtests of the *Bruininks-Oseretsky Test* and the *Body Skills* curriculum	15
Figure 2.1	Developmental sequence for horizontal jumping	17
Figure 2.2	*Body Skills* activity card	19
Figure 2.3	Materials list for Horizontal Jump Activity 2, "Jump and Fetch"	20
Figure 2.4	Preparation section of Horizontal Jump Activity 2	21
Figure 2.5	Individual Skill Checklist	24
Figure 2.6	Class Record Form for locomotor skills	25
Figure 2.7	Lesson plan for using two *Body Skills* activities in a 30-minute lesson	26
Figure 2.8	Example of a two-month calendar from a yearly plan using the *Body Skills* curriculum	27
Figure 3.1	Assessment-intervention system for the *Body Skills* curriculum	31
Figure 3.2	Structure of the *Bruininks-Oseretsky Test of Motor Proficiency*	33
Figure 3.3	MSI Record Booklet Student Achievement Profile	35
Figure 3.4	Sample skill section for stationary balance items from MSI Record Booklet	36
Figure 3.5	Summary of *Bruininks-Oseretsky Test* scores	38
Figure 3.6	*Bruininks-Oseretsky Test* scores plotted on the MSI profile	38
Figure 3.7	*Bruininks-Oseretsky Test* scores, showing standard errors of measurement, on the MSI profile	39
Figure 3.8	Expected range of performance on MSI body management items based on the *Bruininks-Oseretsky Test* Gross Motor Composite score	40
Figure 3.9	Expected range of performance on MSI items based on *Bruininks-Oseretsky Test* Gross Motor Composite and Fine Motor Composite scores	41
Figure 3.10	Sample module section from MSI Record Booklet	42
Figure 3.11	Locomotor profile from MSI Record Booklet	43
Figure 3.12	Completed Class Record Form for locomotor skills	44
Figure 3.13	Completed Individual Educational Planning Form	45
Figure 3.14	*Bruininks-Oseretsky Test Individual Record Form* for Miguel Arroyo	48
Figure 3.15	MSI results for Miguel Arroyo	49
Figure 3.16	MSI profile showing student's performance on locomotor skills before and after instruction	51
Figure 3.17	Class Record Form showing progress on body fitness skills	52
Figure 3.18	MSI profile showing pretest and posttest scores for the *Bruininks-Oseretsky Test* and the MSI	53

Figure 3.19 Individual Skill Checklist showing student's progress 54
Figure 3.20 Student attitude questionnaire 56
Figure 4.1 Procedural model followed for development of the *Body Skills* curriculum 61
Figure 4.2 Field-test evaluation form 69

Tables

Table 3.1 Standard Errors of Measurement for *Bruininks-Oseretsky Test* Point Scores 39
Table 3.2 Recommended *Bruininks-Oseretsky Test* Scores Used to Predict MSI Performance 39
Table 5.1 Equating Study Sample 73
Table 5.2 Kuder-Richardson 20 Reliabilities for MSI Item Clusters 74
Table 5.3 Interrater Reliability Statistics for MSI Module Raw Scores ... 75
Table 5.4 Correlation Between MSI Module Scores and Age 75
Table 5.5 Correlation Between MSI Modules and *Bruininks-Oseretsky Test* Scores 76
Table 5.6 Intercorrelations Among MSI Module Raw Scores 76

Acknowledgments

Completing the *Body Skills* curriculum and the Motor Skills Inventory was facilitated by the contributions of several people.

Early in the development of *Body Skills*, Jeanmarie Pehl assisted by conducting research on the development of motor skills in young children and on existing curricula and instructional techniques. Ms. Pehl made other valuable contributions through the initial development and organization of materials and provided assistance during the field tests and equating study.

Our appreciation is extended to Dr. Heather MacGowan, who ably conducted the first field test of the activities with students in the Osseo, Bloomington, and White Bear school districts in Minnesota.

Important contributions were made by the conscientious teachers in California, Minnesota, and Texas who participated in the second field test.

A special thank you is extended to members of the Minnesota Developmental/Adaptive Physical Education Committee and other physical educators who assisted both in the field testing of activities and in the administration of the tests for the equating study.

Assistance and direction in the conduct of the equating study, analysis of results, preparation of the MSI scoring profiles, and editorial contributions in the preparation of the final manuscripts were made by Kathy Steffens from the University of Minnesota.

Valuable statistical assistance in the calibration and scaling of the items in the equating study was provided by Bob Semmes from the University of Minnesota.

Many schools provided valuable time and assistance to research the *Body Skills* program. This effort could not have been completed without their generous help.

Judy K. Werder
Robert H. Bruininks

January 1988

Chapter 1

Introduction

Motor development plays an important role in cognitive, affective, and physical development of the individual. The study of motor development among children has provided a foundation for developing motor training programs, with many special adaptations for individuals with handicaps and disabilities. Although the scope and content of the total education program for students with handicaps may vary, motor skill training is now considered an integral component of all effective, comprehensive special and general education programs. Special motor training programs can be found within general and adaptive physical education programs, in classrooms, in special schools, and in early childhood programs. Unfortunately, there are few available resource materials that emphasize carefully researched developmental progressions of motor skills among children and youth.

Body Skills: A Motor Development Curriculum for Children is a comprehensive curriculum based on the general pattern of motor skill development in children from two to 12 years of age. The *Body Skills* curriculum provides a systematic method for assessing, planning, and teaching gross motor skills in body management, locomotion, body fitness, and object movement, and fine motor skills. It is useful for special education, adaptive and regular physical education, early childhood and elementary education, and community recreation programs.

Body Skills activities may be used with classes of 15 to 30 students, with smaller groups, and with individual students. In addition, suggested adaptations, variations, and individual practice exercises provide a way for teachers to adapt regular developmental activities to include students with handicapping conditions.

Features

The *Body Skills* program provides the following features:

Instructional Activities. The *Body Skills* program provides a comprehensive curriculum of activities to teach 31 gross and fine motor skills to children and youth. Activities in the program are organized into instructional modules. Figure 1.1 lists the five modules and the motor skills included in each one.

MODULES	BODY MANAGEMENT	LOCOMOTOR	BODY FITNESS	OBJECT MOVEMENT	FINE MOTOR
SKILLS	Body-Space Awareness Moving Balance Stationary Balance Body Rolling Agility	Crawl Walk Horizontal Jump Vertical Jump Run Hop Gallop Skip	Arm-Shoulder Flexibility Midbody Flexibility Aerobic Development Abdominal Strength Leg-Hip Flexibility Leg-Hip Strength Arm-Shoulder Strength	Kick Bounce Catch Overhand Throw Strike Underhand Throw Underhand Roll	Small-Object Control Grasp Hand Strength Visual-Motor Control

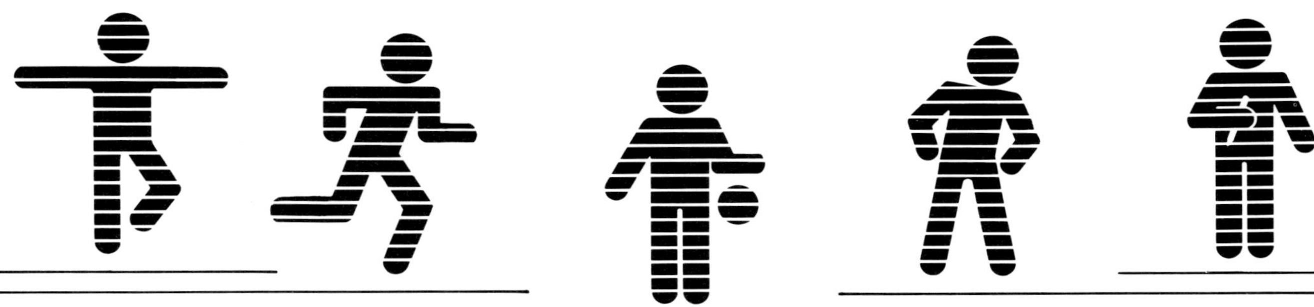

Figure 1.1. Overview of the *Body Skills* curriculum

Assessment. The *Body Skills* program includes an optional assessment component; the curriculum activities may be used without formal assessment. The Motor Skills Inventory (MSI), described in Chapter 3, offers criterion-referenced assessment for measuring a student's current developmental level in the motor skills taught in the *Body Skills* curriculum. Results from administering the MSI are useful in planning and selecting teaching activities. The MSI Record Booklet includes a comprehensive profile which may be used in students' cumulative progress records. A unique feature of the *Body Skills* curriculum is that test results from a standardized measure, the *Bruininks-Oseretsky Test of Motor Proficiency* (Bruininks 1978) can be translated into levels of performance on the MSI, thus providing a direct link to the *Body Skills* teaching activities.

Record-Keeping Forms. Blackline masters for monitoring individual and class progress and for planning are included with the *Body Skills* curriculum.

Organization

Before beginning to use the *Body Skills* curriculum, it is important to become familiar with the materials and format, the skill sequence, and the assessment system.

Materials

The *Body Skills* program is housed in an easy-to carry, portable box that includes:

One *Manual* that contains background information and general instructions, directions for administering and scoring the Motor Skills Inventory (MSI), suggestions for planning and evaluating a physical education program, and information for adapting physical education activities for students with specific handicapping conditions.

Thirty-one *Skill Folders.* Each folder contains illustrations showing the developmental sequence for the skill at a rudimentary, functional, and mature level, the characteristics of each level, background information about the skill, and adaptations for students with handicapping conditions. The skill folders are color-coded by module.

One *Management Folder,* which contains an overview of the *Body Skills* modules and skills, is included for storing the blackline masters.

Two hundred one *Activities.* Five to nine activities are included for each of the skills taught in the *Body Skills* program. Each activity includes the skill objective, a description of the activity, the materials needed, and complete instructions for conducting the activity. In addition, each activity card includes variations for controlling the difficulty of the activity and suggestions for practicing the skill with individual students. The cards are printed back to back (103 cards) and are color-coded by module. The activity cards may be stored in the skill folders in the *Body Skills* box.

Thirty-five *blackline masters,* suitable for reproduction, are included. Seven of the masters are record-keeping forms, and 28 are design sheets used with the fine motor activities.

One *Motor Skills Inventory (MSI) Record Booklet* is included with the *Body Skills* program. The record booklet is used to record an individual student's performance on the MSI, and provides a profile of the student's overall motor skill achievement. Additional MSI record booklets may be purchased in packages of 25.

Scope and Structure of the *Body Skills* Curriculum

Body Skills provides a comprehensive curriculum of activities to teach gross and fine motor skills to children and youth. Following is a brief description of each of the five modules and the 31 skills included in the *Body Skills* curriculum.

Body Management Skills

The Body Management Module includes activities for developing and improving the ability to move one's body in space. This module includes the following five skills:

Body-Space Awareness. Body-space awareness is an individual's awareness of her or his body parts and how to move them in space. Five activities provide opportunities for students to identify body parts and to explore directionality.

Moving Balance. Moving, or dynamic, balance is maintaining one's balance while moving through space; six activities provide opportunities for students to practice balancing their bodies in different positions while moving.

Stationary Balance. Stationary, or static, balance is taught through six activities that lead students from two- and three-point balances to a one-point balance (stork stand) with the eyes closed.

Body Rolling. Six activities provide opportunities for students to practice rocking back and forth and to roll their bodies sideways, backward, and forward.

Agility. Six activities develop agility through a sequence of starting, stopping, dodging, twisting, and turning movements.

Locomotor Skills

The Locomotor Module provides opportunities for students to practice and improve skill in moving one's body forward and upward. This module includes the following eight skills:

Crawling. Six activities emphasize basic crawling movements and arm-leg opposition.

Walking. Six activities emphasize a mature walking pattern.

Horizontal Jumping. Eight activities emphasize a mature horizontal (forward) jump, often called a broad jump.

Vertical Jumping. Six activities emphasize the essential movements of a mature vertical (upward) jump.

Running. Eight activities emphasize mature running.

Hopping. Eight activities emphasize the essential movements of mature hopping on one foot.

Galloping. Six activities provide opportunities for students to develop coordinated galloping movements.

Skipping. Six activities develop ability to move both sides of the body in a mature skipping pattern.

Body Fitness Skills
The Body Fitness Module includes activities for developing and improving the strength, flexibility, and endurance of particular muscle groups of the body. They are divided into the following seven areas:

Arm-Shoulder Flexibility. Five activities feature exercises that require movement of the shoulder joint to improve flexibility.

Midbody Flexibility. Six activities feature twisting and bending movements of the trunk region of the body to improve flexibility.

Aerobic Development. Six activities feature exercises that improve cardiovascular endurance.

Abdominal Strength. Six activities feature exercises that improve the strength of the stomach muscles.

Leg-Hip Flexibility. Six activities feature exercises that require movement of the hip joint to improve flexibility.

Leg-Hip Strength. Six activities feature exercises that improve the muscle strength in the calves, thighs, and hips.

Arm-Shoulder Strength. Six activities feature exercises that improve the muscle strength in the arms and shoulders.

Object Movement Skills
The Object Movement Module includes activities for developing skills in moving an object such as a ball or beanbag. This module includes the following seven skills:

Kicking. Eight activities develop moving balance, leg strength, and eye-foot coordination.

Bouncing and Dribbling. Eight activities progress from bouncing and trapping a ball against the body to stationary dribbling and dribbling while moving.

Catching. Nine activities feature catching a ball in both hands and progress from trapping the ball against the body to catching it with arms extended away from the body.

Overhand Throwing. Nine activities provide practice in developing the essential movements of a mature overhand throw.

Striking. Five activities feature batting a ball or other object and progress from batting a ball from a tee to batting pitched balls.

Underhand Throwing. Six activities feature throwing a palm-sized ball or a beanbag in a mature underhand pattern.

Underhand Rolling. Six activities progress from rolling a ball with both hands to rolling with one hand.

Fine Motor Skills
Four important fine motor skills are included in the *Body Skills* curriculum. In contrast to the skills taught in the first four modules, these skills involve developing the fine muscle groups in the hand, wrist, and arm, and eye-hand

coordination. The activities in this module are most appropriate for use with young children in classroom settings:

Small-Object Control. Six activities give students practice picking up and moving different types of small objects.

Grasping. Eight activities provide opportunities for students to learn to grasp a variety of small objects.

Hand Strength. Six activities encourage students to use only the small muscles of the hand, primarily by squeezing an object.

Visual-Motor Control. Six activities help students develop skill in tracing, copying, and drawing designs, letters, and words.

Body Skills Assessment System

The Motor Skills Inventory (MSI) included in the *Body Skills* curriculum may be given before instruction to help in identifying the modules and skills that need attention. The MSI was developed to provide a means for teachers to measure motor skills in a simple, criterion-referenced format that can be used continuously throughout the school year. It measures qualitative performance of many everyday motor skills. The structure of the MSI corresponds to the organization of activities in the *Body Skills* curriculum—test items are organized into the five skill areas: Body Management, Locomotor, Body Fitness, Object Movement, and Fine Motor. Figure 1.2 shows the number of items on the MSI for each of the modules.

Module	Number of MSI Items
Body Management	15
Locomotor	21
Body Fitness	18
Object Movement	21
Fine Motor	11

Figure 1.2. Organization and content of the Motor Skills Inventory (MSI)

Each skill is divided into three levels of performance:

Rudimentary, in which the basic movements are performed but in an awkward, uncoordinated manner.

Functional, in which the movements are performed adequately but are still slightly awkward.

Mature, in which the movements are performed in a smooth, coordinated manner.

The *Body Skills* curriculum and the MSI together give teachers a means of correlating assessment with instruction by choosing appropriate activities and giving emphasis to the elements of a particular motor skill during instruction. Specific information about administering and scoring the MSI may be found in Chapter 3 and in Appendix A.

The MSI has been statistically equated to the *Bruininks-Oseretsky Test of Motor Proficiency* (Bruininks 1978), a nationally standardized comprehensive motor ability scale. The integration of curriculum-based assessment and motor ability assessment offers unique advantages to users of *Body Skills.*

The *Bruininks-Oseretsky Test* was developed to measure the motor abilities of children and youth, ages 4½ to 14½ years. Because the *Bruininks-Oseretsky Test* was nationally standardized and yields derived scores, it is useful in measuring underlying motor ability comparatively for the purpose of making placement and initial programming decisions. It also helps to pinpoint areas of motor ability in which the student has strengths and weaknesses.

The relationship between the content of the *Bruininks-Oseretsky Test* and the *Body Skills* curriculum is shown in Figure 1.3.

Bruininks-Oseretsky Test Subtests	*Body Skills Curriculum*
Running Speed and Agility	Body Management, Locomotor Skills
Balance	Body Management Skills
Bilateral Coordination	Locomotor Skills
Strength	Body Fitness Skills
Upper-Limb Coordination	Object Movement Skills
Response Speed	Fine Motor Skills
Visual-Motor Control	Fine Motor Skills
Upper-Limb Speed and Dexterity	Fine Motor Skills

Figure 1.3. Relationship between subtests of the *Bruininks-Oseretsky Test* and the *Body Skills* curriculum

Applications

The *Body Skills* curriculum is flexible to meet the needs of a variety of teaching situations. The activities provide specific instructions for teaching each motor skill, as well as a number of ways each activity can be modified to particular teaching situations. The space and equipment requirements for each activity were made as flexible as possible to meet a wide range of settings and equipment. A diagram is included on each activity card to provide an overview of the arrangement of students and equipment. The materials needed for the activities are typical physical education items found in most schools.

The *Body Skills* activities may be used with 15 to 30 students, with smaller groups, and for practice with individual students. Teachers may select activities to match their teaching objectives. The adaptations, activity variations, and suggestions for practice with individual students make it possible for teachers to accommodate the needs of students with handicapping conditions.

The materials included in the *Body Skills* curriculum are designed to be portable and convenient to use. The skill folders and activity cards are printed on durable cards; their format and organization make them convenient to use in nearly any setting.

Regular physical education teachers may integrate the activities into their weekly, monthly, or yearly instructional calendar for each grade level or group. If a yearly schedule is already in place, the curriculum can be used as an activity resource, from which activities may be incorporated into the schedule to meet specified objectives. The flexibility of the *Body Skills* program allows physical education teachers to use the activities to meet their needs, whether physical education is taught on a daily or on a less frequent basis.

Classroom teachers may use the *Body Skills* activities themselves or work with physical education specialists to develop lesson plans. The illustrations and information on the skill folders and the activity cards will help teachers present the activities effectively with a minimum of preparation. Since classroom teachers must be prepared to teach many subjects every day, this program helps reduce precious planning time and ensures that important motor skills will be taught with sound educational principles and instructional methods.

Adaptive physical education teachers may select from a variety of instructional alternatives provided with the *Body Skills* activities. The introductory section of each skill folder provides guidelines for adapting the activities for teaching students with handicapping conditions. Each activity card includes variations for regulating the difficulty of the activity. Additional guidelines for adapting activities for students with specific handicapping conditions are addressed in Appendix B of this manual. By examining the activity itself, the adaptations for students with handicaps, the activity variations, and the options for individual skill practice, the adaptive physical educator will have a number of instructional alternatives for each motor skill.

Early childhood and special education teachers will find many activities that are ideal for use in their programs. Since the *Body Skills* program presents the most elementary or rudimentary levels to more advanced levels of each gross and fine motor skill, the curriculum is useful from the time young children begin to crawl or to grasp objects. The illustrations and the descriptions on the module folders clearly define each level of the motor skills included in the program, and help the nonmotor specialist to become an acute observer and recorder of children's movements.

Occupational therapists and other developmental specialists may use the MSI and the *Body Skills* curriculum to guide teachers in selecting activities appropriate for young children with special needs.

Chapter 2

Using the Body Skills *Curriculum*

This chapter includes general information for using the *Body Skills* activities and provides guidelines for developing lesson plans to implement the activities.

Skill Folders and Activity Cards

Skill Folders

Each of the *Body Skills* modules includes a set of color-coded skill folders. The skills for each module are generally presented in order of increasing difficulty. For example, crawling is the first locomotor skill, and skipping is the last one. The front of each folder identifies the module and skill and has three illustrations with brief descriptions explaining the developmental sequence for that skill. Figure 2.1 shows the developmental sequence for horizontal jumping.

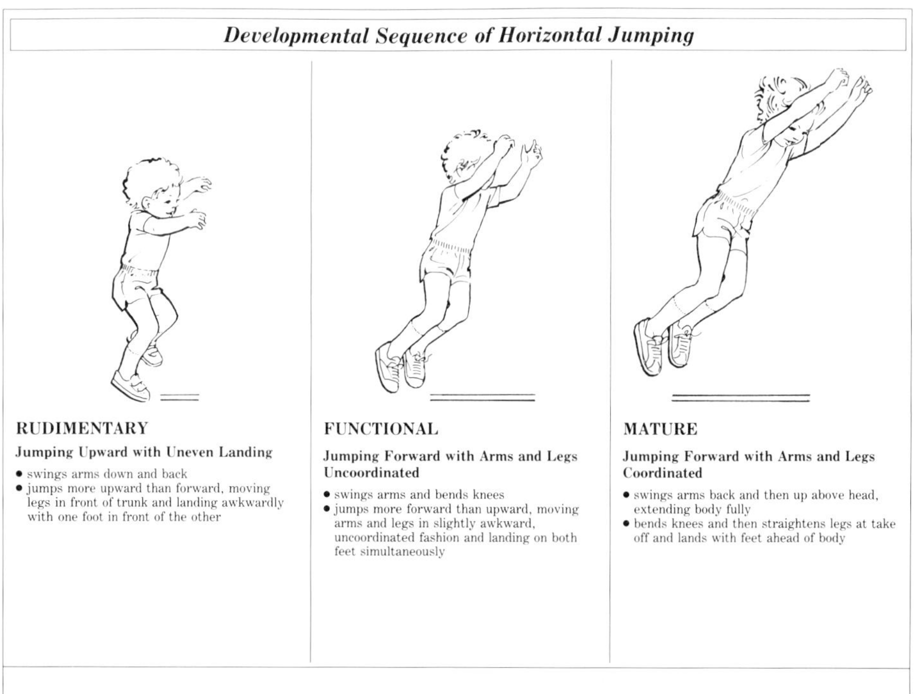

Figure 2.1. Developmental sequence for horizontal jumping

The three developmental levels presented on the folders for each of the motor skills correspond to the items on the Motor Skills Inventory (MSI). Because the MSI and the *Body Skills* curriculum emphasize improving the quality of skill performance, the illustrations and descriptions of the developmental levels are essential to understanding the normal changes in skill performance that occur as children mature and develop proficiency. The three developmental levels for each skill are also important to master for teaching the curriculum activities.

The skills shown in the developmental sequences are usually the same as the actions performed in the related activities. However, for some skills, such as arm-shoulder flexibility, the skill shown (making arm circles) is a representative example of an exercise that requires arm-shoulder flexibility. In this case, the activities for the skill contribute to arm-shoulder flexibility using a number of different exercises. This is true for activities in the Body Management, Body Fitness, and Fine Motor Modules.

Background information about the skill is included on the back of each skill folder, along with suggestions for adapting the activities for students with handicapping conditions. Adaptations of instructional procedures and the environment are included for visually or hearing-impaired students, nonambulatory physically impaired students and students with heart-lung disabilities, ambulatory physically-impaired students with assistive devices, and learning-disabled students. Additional information about adapting the *Body Skills* curriculum for students with handicapping conditions is provided in Appendix B of this manual.

A brief description of the physical setting needed for the activities, and the activity numbers and titles, are also included on the skill folders.

It is recommended that teachers read carefully the introduction to each skill before presenting the instructional activities, paying particular attention to the developmental sequence.

The skill folders and activity cards are color-coded by module as follows:

- Body Management—Green
- Locomotor—Blue
- Body Fitness—Red
- Object Movement—Purple
- Fine Motor—Orange

Activity Cards

Five to nine *Body Skills* activities are included for teaching or reinforcing each skill; a total of 201 instructional activities. These activities provide instruction and practice in the 31 gross and fine motor skills in the curriculum (see Figure 1.1). Each activity includes a number of variations as well as suggestions for practicing the skill with individual students. A complete list of the activities in the *Body Skills* curriculum is provided in Appendix C.

The activities are printed back-to-back on durable cards and color-coded by module. Information at the top of each activity card includes the module and skill name, the activity title, and the activity number (see Figure 2.2). Each activity card also includes:

- Objective
- Time needed
- Materials needed
- Teaching points
- Preparation, including activity set-up diagram
- Directions for conducting the activity
- Variations
- Individual practice suggestions

Locomotor / HORIZONTAL JUMP — ACTIVITY 2

Jump and Fetch

Objective **To practice and improve horizontal-jumping skill.**
In this activity, students compete in a relay race in which they take turns jumping to a finish line, picking up a beanbag, and jumping back.

Time 10 minutes

Materials
- beanbags, one for each student
- floor tape

Teaching Points
- swing arms back and then up above the head
- bend knees and then straighten legs at takeoff
- land with feet ahead of body

Preparation Use the floor tape to make a line at each end of the activity area. Place beanbags behind one of the lines.

Have the students form groups of four or five. Have the groups line up single file behind the starting line, as shown.

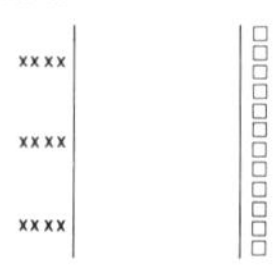

Directions When students are ready, explain that this is a jumping game. Demonstrate a mature horizontal jump as you say: **When you jump, swing your arms down and back and then forward and up. Jump forward as far as you can, bending your knees as you jump. Land on both feet at the same time.**

Then say: **At the signal, the first person in each group will jump to the other line, pick up a beanbag, and jump back. With each jump, jump as far as you can. As soon as the first student crosses the starting line with a beanbag, the second student will jump to get a beanbag. Continue taking turns. The first group to have all members return with a beanbag are the jumpers of the day.**

Give a signal to begin. Continue the activity until all students have jumped across and back.

Variations
1. Vary the distance between the lines to accommodate different skill levels.
2. To make the activity more complex, have the students bring back an object of a certain color or number that they must find in a pile of different-colored or -numbered objects.
3. Have the students count and record the number of jumps and total time for each group. Subtract two seconds for each jump taken from the total group time. The group with the lowest time wins. (This will increase students' awareness of time and encourage students to take longer jumps when the activity is repeated.)

Individual Practice
1. To help coordinate arm and leg movements, guide the student's arms as she jumps.
2. Have the student jump in and out of circles on the floor, or over lines, ropes, or hoops.
3. Have the student jump to a circle or square placed just beyond what would be an easy distance for her to jump.

Figure 2.2. *Body Skills* activity card

Objective. The objective for each activity is composed of two parts: the first part indicates the motor skill that is the focus of the activity, and the second part is a brief statement describing the nature of the activity. For example, the objective for Horizontal Jumping Activity 2, "Jump and Fetch":

> *To develop and improve horizontal-jumping skill.*
> *In this activity, students complete a relay race in which they take turns jumping to a finish line, picking up a beanbag, and jumping back.*

Time and Materials. Most of the activities in the *Body Skills* curriculum take about 10 to 15 minutes for a class to perform. The activity time may vary according to the skill, attention span, and energy levels of students in the class. The attention span and the energy levels of students should be monitored, and the activity varied to insure optimum motivation and participation of the students. The activities provide maximum participation of the students from the beginning to the close of the activity rather than having one or two students participate actively while other students watch. Most activities are structured so that all students are practicing the motor skill about 80 to 95 percent of the activity time. In a typical 25-to-30 minute physical education class, two *Body Skills* activities may be taught, providing students with opportunities to learn and improve performance on two objectives during one lesson.

Materials needed to conduct the activity are listed on each activity card (see Figure 2.3). The activities use materials and equipment that are commonly found in physical education departments or elementary school classrooms. Prior to beginning instruction, the materials should be gathered and organized for the activity. Materials frequently used for the gross motor activity modules include rubber activity balls, mats, small foam or yarn balls, floor tape or other material to mark lines on the floor, targets to mount on walls, cones, and musical recordings. Materials may require adaptation to accommodate the needs of students with handicaps. All materials used should be both durable and safe. Safe materials have no sharp edges or appendages, are of appropriate weight for the students, and are kept in good condition. Balls should be inflated appropriately.

Materials	• beanbags, one for each student • floor tape

Figure 2.3. Materials list for Horizontal Jump Activity 2

Teaching Points. While the activities are designed to be enjoyable for students, the primary purpose of the activities is to serve as a vehicle for teaching and providing practice of basic motor skills. Teaching points are provided on each activity card to summarize the essential movements that are characteristic of the mature skill pattern. The teaching points provide guidance for emphasizing components of the mature skill pattern while teaching. For example, the teaching points for horizontal jumping:

- swing arms back and then up above the head
- bend knees and then straighten legs at takeoff
- land with feet ahead of the body

The teaching points reiterate the essential movements in a mature horizontal jump, as evident from the skill description and the illustrated developmental sequence shown on the skill folder. If a student is at the rudimentary level in horizontal jumping, teaching may focus primarily on the upward arm swing, an element missing at this level of performance. With this approach, the teacher may choose to emphasize any of the teaching points that are most needed by the students to eventually achieve a mature horizontal jump. When teaching any of the horizontal jumping activities, the teaching points should be used for guidance when giving verbal directions and when demonstrating the skill. In some cases, such as the Body Fitness activities, the movements used in the activity are not the same as the sequence described on the outside of the folder. In these cases, the activity contributes to the skill development through a different but related motor task, adding variety to the activities.

Preparation. The preparation section includes an illustration of the activity set up and describes the placement of the students and the materials. Each diagram shows the activity set up for 12-15 students. Adjustments for more or fewer students can be made by modifying the group sizes and the number of materials.

For the gross motor modules, the distances are suggested for average-sized gymnasiums and can easily be increased or reduced to suit the needs of the class and the activity area. Figure 2.4 presents the preparation section for Horizontal Jumping Activity 2, "Jump and Fetch."

Preparation Use the floor tape to make a line at each end of the activity area. Place beanbags behind one of the lines.

Have the students form groups of four or five. Have the groups line up single file behind the starting line, as shown.

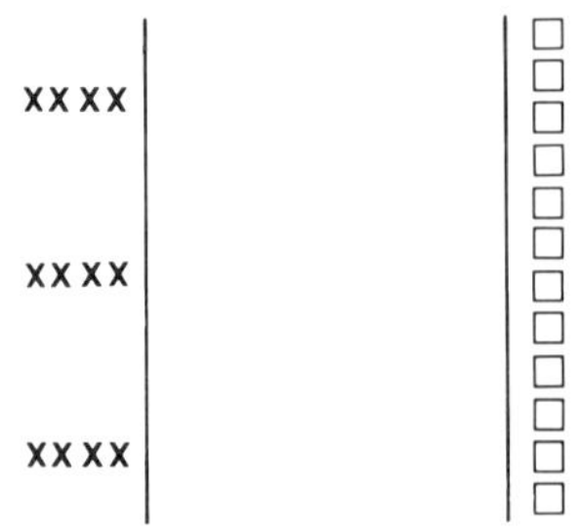

Figure 2.4. Preparation section of Horizontal Jump Activity 2

Directions. The directions for the activity explain what the teacher should do and say to conduct the activity. Verbal directions for teachers to give to students are presented in bold type for emphasis. The activities all begin with verbal directions and a simultaneous teacher demonstration of the mature pattern of the skill. While saying the directions, the teacher, or a model student, should demonstrate the movements. For example, **When you jump, move your arms down and back, then forward and up, and jump as far forward as possible.**

Next, the teacher explains the activity directions to students. Most activities begin with a signal. The signal may be a word, such as "Go," or "Begin," or it may be the sound of a whistle or bell. During the activity, the teacher should be stationed in a position to easily supervise all students. If student attention and energy levels allow, the activity may be repeated once or several times as part of a single lesson.

Variations. Variations of the activity are presented after the directions on each activity card. The variations section provides suggestions for teaching the same activity with minor changes as a means of extending the activity. The variations might include changes in the materials, the distances, and complexity of the activity. When an activity is particularly successful, or when students are in need of further practice in performing a skill, the variations provide many suggestions for extending the curriculum and increasing its flexibility. The variations suggested can be viewed as alternative activities.

Individual Practice. The final section of each activity card provides suggestions for individual practice. The individual practice suggestions are ideal for teachers who have the opportunity to work with individual students in small classes, in adapted physical education classes, or in small groups within a large class. The suggestions include recommendations for helping students on a one-to-one basis, sometimes giving physical guidance for the skill movements.

Teaching the Activities

The *Body Skills* activity cards contain all of the essential information needed to teach the activities; it is recommended that the activity card information be studied prior to instruction. Placing the activity card on a clipboard will keep it handy for easy reference while teaching. The materials should be gathered and arranged according to the diagram on the activity card.

Begin the activity by telling the students that a particular motor skill, like hopping, is the focus of the activity. It is helpful to remind the students verbally and with demonstration how the skill is to be performed during the activity. For example, students may be hopping to get to a goal, and may be excited about not being caught. In their excitement, they may become sloppy or careless about how they hop and forget to concentrate on improving the skill. It is often useful for the teacher to stop the activity between rounds and review the essential movements by demonstrating the mature pattern of the featured skill.

Motivation and reinforcement are key concepts in successful teaching. As students are participating in the activity and demonstrating the skill, it is important to provide feedback. Students should be told when they should reach their arms higher, or when they should watch the ball more closely, and especially, when they are performing the skill well and are following directions. Positive reinforcement helps to make practice an enjoyable growth experience, rather than simply a tedious drill. Praise students by making comments such as: "I like the way you swung your arms way above your head when you jumped"; "Yes, Lisa, keep your eye on the target when you throw"; and "Way to go, Sarah, you really ran a nice even pace." These statements are not only positive, but they also provide specific feedback about the student's correct movements and efforts in relationship to the mature performance standard. For students who are performing the skill incorrectly, feedback can still be positive. For example, the teacher might say: "Jason, you are trying very hard. Now try to roll the ball with both hands, like this" (demonstrate), or "Benjamin, let's try to cross the line by hopping on one foot this time, like this" (demonstrate). It may also be useful to award points to groups for the quality of their performances during the activities.

The general strategy in teaching the activities is to describe the movements while demonstrating the mature performance level. It may be useful to employ some additional teaching strategies:

- Present the specific components of the skill sequentially in small steps. (This is often referred to as a task analysis approach to teaching.) Describing and practicing the component parts of each skill can be a useful, introductory part of each activity.
- As the specific parts of each skill are mastered, provide practice in integrating them into the complete skill movements. Provide continuous, positive feedback to the students as they make progress toward mature performance of a skill.
- Provide manual guidance. For some students, demonstration is more effective when manual guidance is used to gently move the body parts through the skill movement, so that the student gets the "feel" of moving correctly.
- Provide opportunities for students to practice the skill repeatedly. Encourage the students, emphasizing correct movements as needed.
- Encourage the students to verbalize their movements by asking them questions, such as: "What did you do? How did you get to the goal? How can you jump farther?"

Monitoring Progress While Teaching

It is useful to record observations of individual skill performance during or right after an activity or exercise.

The Individual Skill Checklist, included with the *Body Skills* blackline masters, may be used to monitor a student's progress during activities. The student's information, dates, and performance level may be recorded on the sheet, as shown in Figure 2.5.

The checklist master should be duplicated for each student. The date and performance level may be recorded during or right after activities. The checklists will be helpful in choosing skills to review and in planning activities. The checklist provides room to evaluate student progress several different times. It is recommended that student performance be evaluated monthly, if possible.

The Class Record Form, also included with the *Body Skills* blackline masters, can be used to record the performance of all students in a class on the motor skills in each module. Figure 2.6 shows a Class Record Form for locomotor skills.

Items from the Motor Skills Inventory (MSI) can be administered while an activity is in progress or after an activity. This method of observational assessment works best when an initial baseline assessment has already been administered. A teacher could simply record pass (+) or fail (-) on the MSI Record Booklet for the levels of skill development being demonstrated by the student during the activity. Assessing while teaching helps maintain a continuous, up-to-date record of skill performance.

INDIVIDUAL SKILL CHECKLIST

Name *Leah Kocena* Class *Mrs. Erhardt*

Period *1:45 -2:15 MWF* Grade ______ Birthdate *7-3-82*

Instructions: Record the date for each evaluation. For each skill, record an R for *rudimentary* performance, an F for *functional* performance, or an M for *mature* performance.

Date:	9/15				
Body Management					
Body-Space Awareness	M				
Moving Balance	F				
Stationary Balance	M				
Body Roll	R				
Agility	F				
Locomotor					
Crawl	M				
Walk	M				
Horizontal Jump	M				
Vertical Jump	F				
Run	M				
Hop	M				
Gallop	M				
Skip	F				
Body Fitness					
Arm-Shoulder Flexibility	M				
Midbody Flexibility	M				
Aerobic Development	R				
Abdominal Strength	F				
Leg-Hip Flexibility	M				
Leg-Hip Strength	F				
Arm-Shoulder Strength	F				
Object Movement					
Kick	F				
Bounce	F				
Catch	F				
Overhand Throw	R				
Strike	R				
Underhand Throw	F				
Underhand Roll	M				
Fine Motor					
Small-Object Control	M				
Grasp	M				
Hand Strength	M				
Visual-Motor Control	M				

Figure 2.5. Individual Skill Checklist

LOCOMOTOR SKILLS
Class Record Form

Class ______________________________ Period ______________

Instructions: Record the date for each evaluation. For each student, record R for *rudimentary* performance, an F for *functional* performance, or an M for *mature* performance.

Students' Names	Skill:	Crawl	Walk	Horizontal Jump	Vertical Jump	Run	Hop	Gallop	Skip
	Date:								

Figure 2.6. Class Record Form for locomotor skills

Developing Lesson Plans

Body Skills activities take from 10 to 15 minutes for the average class to complete. For longer periods, two activities may be combined to create a 20- to 30-minute lesson plan. Figure 2.7 presents a sample lesson plan combining two different *Body Skills* activities. When selecting activities to combine, the following considerations should be made:

1. Combine activities that teach different skills. By selecting different skills, the teacher will maximize student interest and will prevent fatigue of one part of the body.
2. Combine activities that use the same equipment, or one activity that uses equipment and another that doesn't, so that the lesson doesn't need to be interrupted to rearrange equipment.
3. Combine activities that have different formats. For example, combine a circle formation activity with a relay formation activity. This variation also stimulates student interest.
4. Combine beginning activities from each skill. The first activities for each skill (Activities 1 and 2) generally have a simpler format, strategy, and organization than later activities for that skill. Younger children, or children just beginning a new skill, should be exposed to the earlier activities first, and more advanced activities later. This order is not required, but it is recommended when teaching a skill over several class periods.

Date 10/22/87 Class 2nd. Grade (Brown) Time Period 10:00-10:30
Materials Tape Player, tape, bean bags or blocks, floor tape

Time	Activity	Skill	Comments
10:00-10:05 (5 min.)	Warm up (jogging to music, stretching)		
10:05-10:15 (5 min.)	Activity 2 Roll to Gold Note: Emphasize smooth rolling	Body Rolls	
10:15-10:25 (10 min.)	Activity 2 Side to Side Note: Emphasize keeping hips and legs still	Midbody Flexibility	
10:25-10:30	Cool Down (review skills stretch, relax)		

Figure 2.7. Lesson plan for using two *Body Skills* activities in a 30-minute lesson

5. Select activities that reinforce prior learning. If hopping was taught on Monday, hopping should also be taught on subsequent days. This approach has a spiraling effect by distributing practice and increasing efficiency in learning, so that skills taught for several consecutive weeks can be reinforced later in the school year through the introduction of new activities or with variations of activities taught earlier.
6. Always provide a warm-up period for two to five minutes for students to bring their heart rate up and to stretch their muscles. The flexibility or aerobic activities in the *Body Skills* program may be used as warm-up activities. An introduction to the daily lesson can also be presented during the warm-up. A cool-down period of reviewing skills practiced, of stretching muscles, and relaxing should be included at the end of the session.

Figure 2.8 presents a sample two-month calendar of *Body Skills* activities. A complete annual plan for nine months is included in Appendix D.

october

sunday	monday	tuesday	wednesday	thursday	friday	saturday
				1	2 Arm-Sh Flex 2 Run 4 (Var) Kick 1 (Var)	3
4	5 Arm-Sh Flex 2 (Var) H Jump 1 Kick 2 (Var)	6	7 Arm-Sh Flex 3 H. Jump 1 (Var) Kick 3	8	9 Aerobic Ser 5 H Jump 2 Kick 3 (Var)	10
11	12 Aerobic Ser 6 H Jump 3 Kick 4	13	14 Catch 1 H Jump 4 Kick 4 (Var)	15	16 Catch 2 H Jump 4 (Var) Kick 5	17
18	19 Catch 3 H Jump 5 Kick 5 (Var)	20	21 Catch 4 Leg-Hip Strength 1 Kick 6	22 Conferences	23	24
25	26 Catch 5 Leg-Hip Strength 2 Kick 6 (Var)	27	28 Catch 6 Leg-Hip Strength 3 Hop 1	29	30 Halloween Choice Day	31

november

sunday	monday	tuesday	wednesday	thursday	friday	saturday
1	2 Body Roll 3 Midbody Flex 4 Hop 2	3	4 Body Roll 3 (Var) Bounce 1 Hop 1 (Var)	5	6 Body Roll 4 Bounce 2 Hop 2 (Var)	7
8	9 Bounce 2 (Var) Run 3 Hop 3	10	11 Bounce 3 Run 3 (Var) Hop 3 (Var)	12	13 School Assembly – No Class	14
15	16 Bounce 4 Run 4 Hop 3 (Var)	17	18 Bounce 3 (Var) Run 4 (Var) Hop 4	19	20 Bounce 4 (Var) Run 2 (Var) Hop 4 (Var)	21
22	23 School Assembly No Class	24	25 Agility 1 Arm-Sh Flex 3 (Var) Gallop 1	26 Thanksgiving Holiday	27	28
29	30 Agility 2 Arm-Sh Flex 4 Gallop 2					

Figure 2.8. Example of a two-month calendar from a yearly plan using the *Body Skills* curriculum

Planning a yearly program consists of clearly defining the annual educational goals for students and the requirements of the teaching assignment, and then determining the schedule and lesson plans for achieving those goals. Many states have mandated specific performance objectives in general education, special education, and physical education. After studying state-mandated and school district goals, a complete list of annual physical education goals that apply to all students, including those with disabilities, should be developed. In addition to physical development goals, physical education and other educational programs should provide opportunities for all students to develop skills in cooperation, problem solving, and knowledge of health and fitness.

Planning an Assessment Schedule

Assessment is an essential part of sound teaching. Without assessment, a teacher would be teaching the activity, not the skill underlying the activity, and certainly not at an appropriate level for the students. One of the biggest dilemmas facing teachers is how to assess students individually when they are always faced with teaching a classroom of students. There are several options in scheduling assessments of students.

Assessment can be conducted in the fall to gather information to assist in developing lesson plans. The *Bruininks-Oseretsky Test* (or other tests) or the MSI will provide information about each student's motor proficiency. The *Body Skills* assessment system provides information that can be linked directly to teaching activities in the *Body Skills* program.

Individualized assessment can be done by a specialist outside of the physical education or other classrooms or through a "station approach" during physical education and other classes. A station approach is an organized method of assessment in which certain subtests are assigned to stations established in a gymnasium or an open area. Each station must be managed by a trained aide or teacher who records each student's performance on specific subtest items. The results of these tests administered in the fall can be considered pretests and the same instruments can be readministered in the spring to measure student progress over a one-year period.

Another assessment option is to assess skill areas that correspond to skills being taught just prior to teaching those activities. For example, the MSI items can be easily administered during a class session. With this option, assessment would truly be "curriculum-imbedded" and implemented prior to instruction throughout the school year. This method provides the teacher with current information about the students' skill levels and guides in selecting and teaching activities to meet the skill level needs of the students.

Other ways to assess skills include:

Using the district's performance objectives as test items to discover how students match district criteria.

Using standardized tests to measure the quality of students' motor skill performances. The *Bruininks-Oseretsky Test* may be most beneficial to adaptive physical education teachers who find normative comparisons on motor ability useful, or the *Body Skills* MSI to measure motor skills of individual students without normative comparisons.

This chapter has focused on using *Body Skills* activities, with suggestions for planning lessons, monitoring student progress, and assessment. The MSI is an optional feature of the *Body Skills* program that provides a means for determining students' motor skill performance levels before, during, or following instruction. The next chapter provides information on assessment strategies, using the MSI and the *Bruininks-Oseretsky Test,* that can be used to provide comprehensive information about students' motor abilities and skill performance.

Chapter 3

Assessment, Instructional Planning, and Evaluation

While the *Body Skills* activities may be used without assessment, they can also be used as part of an assessment-intervention process to remediate specific motor skill deficiencies. This chapter presents information on assessment strategies, incorporating the *Bruininks-Oseretsky Test of Motor Proficiency* and the Motor Skills Inventory (MSI), that may be used with the *Body Skills* curriculum. It also provides detailed information on planning and evaluating instruction.

Assessment Strategies

Figure 3.1 describes the assessment-intervention processes that may be used with the *Body Skills* curriculum.

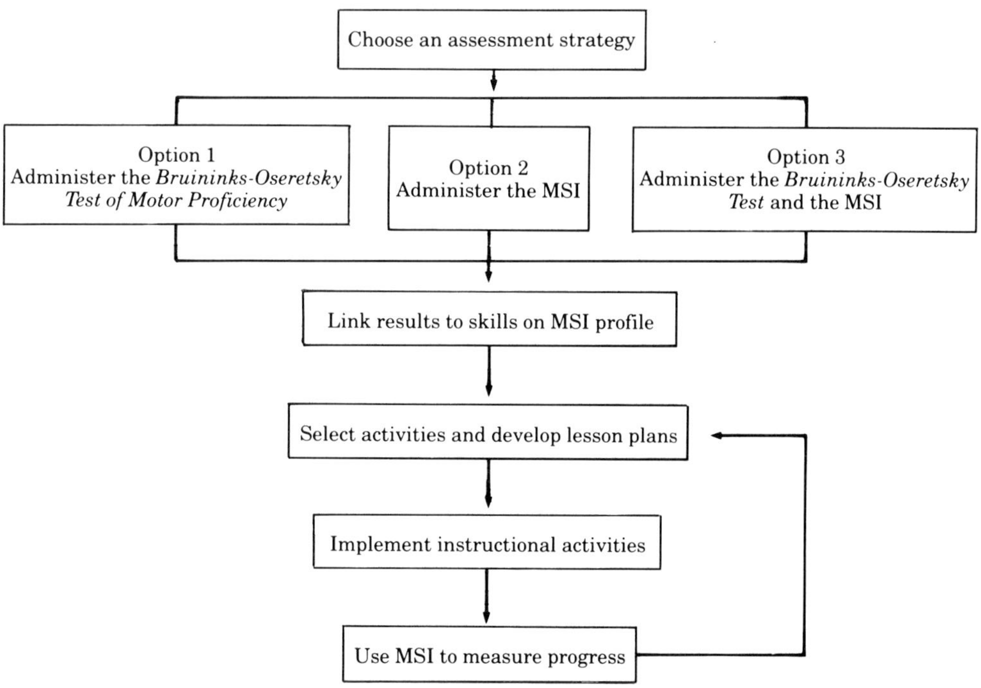

Figure 3.1. Assessment-intervention system for the *Body Skills* curriculum.

The steps depicted in Figure 3.1 portray an integrated approach to assessment, instruction, and evaluation. Three assessment options are available in this program: *Option 1*—administer the *Bruininks-Oseretsky Test*; *Option 2*—administer the MSI; Option 3—administer both the *Bruininks-Oseretsky Test* and the MSI.

In the first option, only the *Bruininks-Oseretsky Test* is administered to students. In many programs, the *Bruininks-Oseretsky Test* is used for initial evaluation to assess the fine and gross motor ability of individual students. This test provides an estimate of the student's motor ability using age-based standardized scores (for example, standard scores, percentile ranks, age scores) that compare the performance to that of a representative norming sample. The *Bruininks-Oseretsky Test* provides a structured, detailed assessment of motor proficiency in eight areas. The test scores have been directly linked to developmental levels of the fundamental motor skills in the *Body Skills* program and the MSI through a special statistical equating study described in Chapter 5.

The second option allows users to enter the program through direct administration of the MSI, or parts of the MSI. The MSI is individually administered; it assesses all the motor skills included in the *Body Skills* program, except crawling, showing at which level of each skill the student is performing.

The third option involves comprehensive assessment of motor ability and skills by administering both the *Bruininks-Oseretsky Test* and the MSI. This option provides the most information about a student's entry level performance or underlying motor ability and fundamental motor skills. The *Bruininks-Oseretsky Test* is administered first, and then the MSI can be used to identify the student's level of performance on specific motor skills.

Whichever option or assessment strategy is used, this phase of the assessment-intervention system provides a foundation for planning instruction and selecting teaching activities from the *Body Skills* program. After assessment, the results may be profiled to provide a clear indication of the developmental status of each individual on the skills taught in *Body Skills*.

Progress in motor skill development can be specifically evaluated at planned intervals during the school year or at the end of the school year through administration of the MSI. These results may be used as a continual evaluation and update of the individual's status or the status of a group in achieving maximum performance on specified motor skills.

The three assessment options all involve individual or combined use of the *Bruininks-Oseretsky Test of Motor Proficiency* and/or the MSI. Following is a brief description of the content and organization of the two tests.

Bruininks-Oseretsky Test of Motor Proficiency. The *Bruininks-Oseretsky Test of Motor Proficiency* assesses the motor functioning of children from 4½ to 14½ years of age. The Complete Battery—eight subtests comprised of 46 separate items—provides a comprehensive index of motor proficiency as well as separate measures of both gross and fine motor abilities. The Short Form—14 items from the Complete Battery—provides a brief survey of general motor proficiency. Administration of the Complete Battery requires about 45-60 minutes; the Short Form requires about 15-20 minutes.

The *Bruininks-Oseretsky Test* was developed to provide educators, clinicians, and researchers with useful information to assist them in assessing the motor abilities of individual students, in developing and evaluating motor training programs, and in assessing serious motor dysfunctions and developmental handicaps in children. Normative data, based on the performance of a carefully selected sample of subjects tested in the standardization program, yield standard scores for each age group, percentile ranks, and stanines. Age equivalents are also provided for each of the eight subtests.

Each of the eight subtests in the *Bruininks-Oseretsky Test* is designed to assess an important aspect of motor ability. Four of the subtests measure gross motor functioning, three measure fine motor functioning, and one measures both gross and fine motor ability. The differentiated measurement of gross and fine motor ability makes it possible to obtain meaningful comparisons of performance in the two areas.

The Complete Battery of the *Bruininks-Oseretsky Test* yields three estimates of motor proficiency: a Gross Motor Composite, a Fine Motor Composite, and a Battery Composite. Figure 3.2 shows the eight subtests and their relationship to the composites.

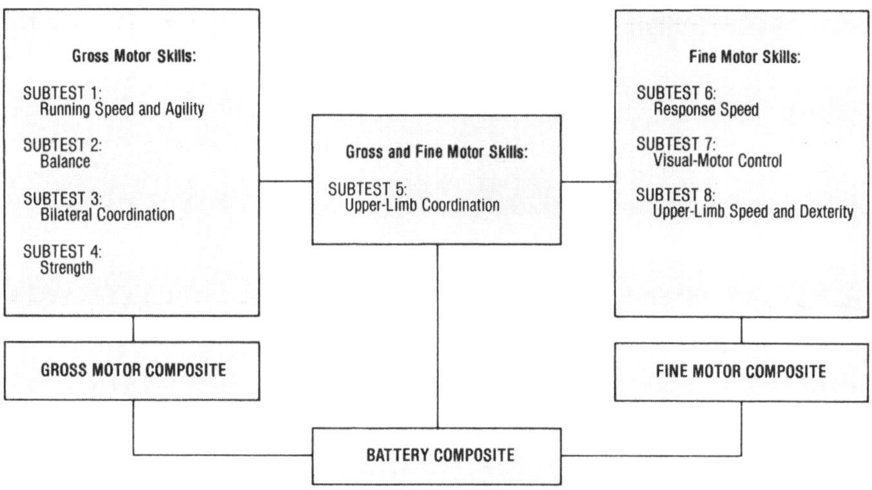

Figure 3.2. Structure of the *Bruininks-Oseretsky Test of Motor Proficiency.* Reprinted from the *Bruininks-Oseretsky Test of Motor Proficiency Examiner's Manual* (©1978 by American Guidance Service, Inc.).

The Short Form of the *Bruininks-Oseretsky Test* is designed for use in situations that require only a brief survey of general motor proficiency. A single score provides an index of general motor proficiency. The Short Form provides a quick assessment and may be used when large numbers of children must be tested in a limited amount of time.

Administration of either form of the *Bruininks-Oseretsky Test* is a helpful first step in selecting priorities for using the *Body Skills* program. The user can start by examining the pattern of performance across subtests and battery scores (Gross Motor, Fine Motor, Short Form, Total Battery), looking for areas that are seriously below average for age or seriously low compared to a subject's other areas of performance. With completion of the *Bruininks-Oseretsky Test*, the user can plot the scores on the profile on the back of the MSI Record Booklet and use the scores to select specific *Body Skills* activities that address skill areas needing improvement. Specific guidelines and an outline of procedural steps for converting scores from the *Bruininks-Oseretsky Test* into the skill levels of fundamental motor movements of the MSI are provided in the next section of this chapter.

MSI. The MSI, included with the *Body Skills* curriculum, is a curriculum-based measure. It assesses a student's performance level for 29 of the 30 skills taught in *Body Skills*. (The MSI does not assess crawling, and the same MSI items are used to assess vertical jumping and leg-hip strength.) The skills are classified into five categories that represent broad areas of motor development for children and youth and correlate with the five modules in the *Body Skills* curriculum. The five categories and specific skill areas are shown in Figure 1.1.

Each of the 29 skills assessed by the MSI is divided into three developmental achievement levels that assess the quality of the student's performance.

> *Rudimentary*. At this early stage of skill development, the individual can do only parts of the movement or skill, does the tasks very awkwardly, and does not integrate movements in a coordinated manner.
>
> *Functional*. At this level, most of the movements of the skill can be performed, but the movements have not been mastered or integrated into a smoothly performed motor pattern. The task can be performed, but not well.
>
> *Mature*. At this level, all the component movements are performed in a well-integrated and coordinated fashion.

Nearly all items on the MSI assess the quality of performance. However, items in the Body Fitness Module require a standard of performance be met at each level. For example, mature performance for arm-shoulder strength requires continuous push-ups for 20 seconds.

For each item, the examiner marks the level that best describes the quality of the student's performance. Performance on the MSI is evaluated in relationship to individual skills, and it does not produce total module or test scores. Normative development of motor skills must be assessed by the *Bruininks-Oseretsky Test* or by some other appropriate standardized measure.

Instructions for administering and scoring the MSI are in Appendix A of this manual. The Record Booklet is an eight-page response booklet for recording performance in five broad motor skill areas. A special profile appears on the back cover of the record booklet for marking the individual performance levels for the MSI motor skills (see Figure 3.3). This profile also includes a place to record *Bruininks-Oseretsky Test* scores.

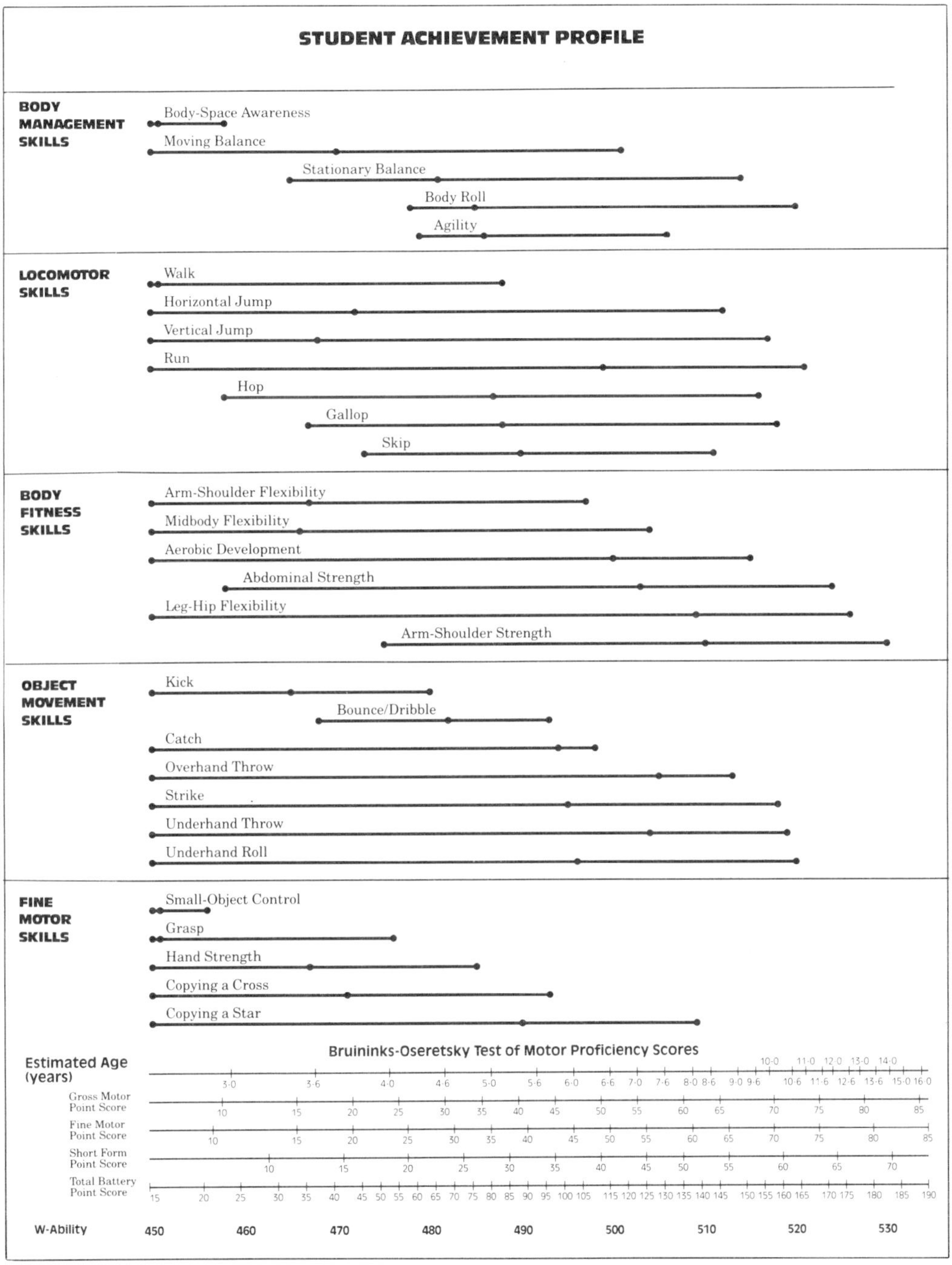

Figure 3.3. MSI Record Booklet Student Achievement Profile

Instructions for the MSI

Detailed information on the administration and scoring of the MSI is included in Appendix A of this manual. The MSI assesses a subject's developmental level of fundamental childhood motor skills. Each skill is classified into one of five areas (modules) and evaluated by developmental levels. The subject is usually given up to three trials to pass a skill level. The examiner administers each skill according to the standard instructions in Appendix A and observes the performance in relationship to the scoring criteria. Scores are recorded as plus (+) for pass and minus (-) for fail for each level of the skill. When the student achieves a plus, for mature performance, the examiner stops administering that skill and goes on to the next skill.

The instructions in Appendix A should be read carefully before administering the MSI. Following are some general guidelines.

1. Some items are marked with an asterisk (*). To save testing time, examiners should begin with the marked (*) item. If the subject passes that item, plusses should be given for all lower levels of performance for the same skill. If the subject fails the marked item, the lower levels should be administered and scored.
2. Student performance for each skill should be carefully observed to ensure that all movements for the particular skill level are performed correctly before awarding credit for passing it.
3. Students are allowed up to three trials to pass each item. The objective is to assess the individual's best level of performance. If a student displays the highest (mature) level of performance on the first trial, the student should be given a plus for the mature level.

Stationary Balance

RUDIMENTARY	Standing on one leg for five seconds with eyes open		___ seconds	+
*FUNCTIONAL	Standing on one leg for ten seconds with eyes open		10 seconds	+
MATURE	Standing on one leg for ten seconds with eyes closed	6 5 (8)	8 seconds	−

Figure 3.4. Sample skill section for stationary balance items from MSI Record Booklet

Figure 3.4 presents a sample illustration of the administration sequence for the stationary balance items in the MSI. The examiner begins by administering the marked item. The student performed the skill correctly in ten seconds, thus was given a passing score for that item and for the preceding item. Then the next item (mature) was administered, and the student did not meet the performance criteria on the first trial. Two more trials were administered, and the student balanced on one leg, eyes closed, for eight seconds on the third trial. The third trial was the student's best performance, so the eight seconds and a minus were recorded in the Record Booklet. No more trials for a skill should be administered when the student performs the item correctly at the highest mature level. Unless the directions specifically require that the skill be performed with less than three trials, the recommended number of trials should be allowed.

The MSI primarily assesses the quality of an individual's performance in relationship to criteria that have been arranged in a developmental hierarchy. Correct scoring depends upon the examiner's observation and judgment in relationship to the scoring criteria.

Interpreting Assessment Results for Instructional Planning

This section presents a step-by-step guide for interpreting results from the *Bruininks-Oseretsky Test* and the MSI into teaching plans. It is useful to refer to the *Individual Record Form* of the *Bruininks-Oseretsky Test* and the MSI Record Booklet in reading this material.

Step 1: Administer and score the *Bruininks-Oseretsky Test.* To convert performance on the *Bruininks-Oseretsky Test* to a prediction of likely performance on the MSI requires only a few simple procedures. First, the user must decide whether to administer the Gross Motor Battery Subtests, the Fine Motor Battery Subtests, the Total Battery, or the Short Form. The example presented in Figure 3.5 shows the results of administering the Total Battery, as well as the Short Form score. To complete the MSI Profile (in Step 2), please note that the point scores for subtests are totaled for each composite, a minor variation in the usual *Bruininks-Oseretsky Test* scoring procedure. The point scores of Subtests 1-4 are totaled to derive the Gross Motor Battery Composite, resulting in a score of 41. The point scores for Subtests 6, 7, and 8 are totaled to derive the Fine Motor Battery Composite score of 30. The point scores for the Total Battery Composite, the sum of all eight subtests, is 79. Only the point scores are used in converting the *Bruininks-Oseretsky Test* scores to a predicted range of MSI skills performance. In either Option 1 or Option 3, the user is advised to use normative scores provided by the *Bruininks-Oseretsky Test* in the process of determining comparative strengths and weaknesses in motor ability and eligibility for program placement.

Step 2: Convert *Bruininks-Oseretsky Test* scores into predicted performance on the MSI skill items. The next task is to mark an (X) corresponding to the point scores obtained on the *Bruininks-Oseretsky Test* on the bottom portion of the profile found on the back page of the MSI Record Booklet (see Figure 3.6). If the Total Gross Motor and Fine Motor Batteries had been administered, the plot would not include the Short Form score.

Step 3: Estimate performance ranges for the MSI from *Bruininks-Oseretsky Test* scores. This step involves using the *Bruininks-Oseretsky Test* scores to estimate the range of performance on the MSI skills. To accomplish this task, it is desirable to portray the *Bruininks-Oseretsky Test* scores in performance ranges. This is accomplished by marking a range above and below the score using the Standard Errors of Measurement for the *Bruininks-Oseretsky Test* in Table 3.1. The standard errors of measurement reflect the expected variation around an individual's score if he or she were to take the test repeatedly. All of us would produce some variation in our performance on different days or at different times. This statistic is a convenient way to illustrate such expected variation in the performance of individuals on the same measure.

Please note that Table 3.1 provides estimates from the equating research sample for ±1 and ±2 standard errors of measurement. A description of the equating study is included in Chapter 5. At ±1 standard error of measurement, it is expected that these score limits would include the individual's test performance about 68 percent of the time. An individual's score would be expected to fall between ±2 standard errors of measurement 95 percent of the time. For maximum confidence, it is recommended that users plot the range of *Bruininks-Oseretsky Test* scores using ±2 standard errors of measurement about the individual's score.

Complete Battery:

SUBTEST	POINT SCORE Maximum	POINT SCORE Subject's	STANDARD SCORE Test (Table 23)	STANDARD SCORE Composite (Table 24)	PERCENTILE RANK (Table 25)	STANINE (Table 25)	OTHER
GROSS MOTOR SUBTESTS:							
1. Running Speed and Agility	15	5					
2. Balance	32	10					
3. Bilateral Coordination	20	8					
4. Strength	42	18					
GROSS MOTOR COMPOSITE		41	* SUM				
5. Upper-Limb Coordination	21	8	*				
FINE MOTOR SUBTESTS:							
6. Response Speed	17	8					
7. Visual-Motor Control	24	6					
8. Upper-Limb Speed and Dexterity	72	16					
FINE MOTOR COMPOSITE		30	* SUM				
BATTERY COMPOSITE		79	* SUM				

*To obtain Battery Composite: Add Gross Motor Composite, Subtest 5 Standard Score, and Fine Motor Composite. Check result by adding Standard Scores on Subtests 1-8.

Short Form:

	POINT SCORE Maximum	POINT SCORE Subject's	STANDARD SCORE (Table 27)	PERCENTILE RANK (Table 27)	STANINE (Table 27)
SHORT FORM	98	26			

Figure 3.5. Summary of *Bruininks-Oseretsky Test* scores. Individual Record Form reprinted from *Bruininks-Oseretsky Test of Motor Proficiency* (©1978 by American Guidance Service, Inc.)

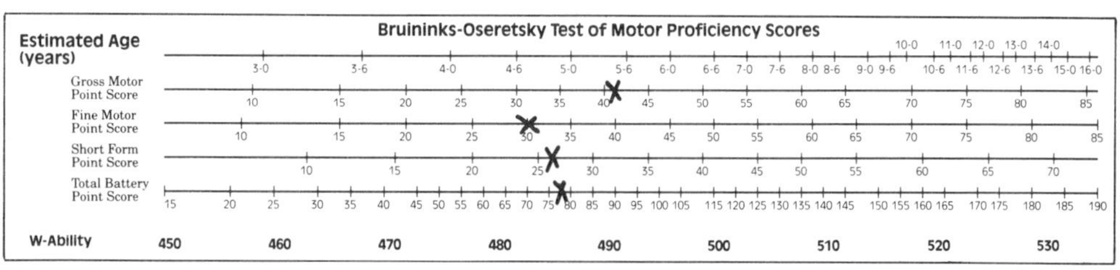

Figure 3.6. *Bruininks-Oseretsky Test* scores plotted on the MSI profile

Table 3.1
Standard Errors of Measurement
for *Bruininks-Oseretsky Test* Point
Scores[a]

Score	1-SEM	2-SEM
Gross Motor Composite	3.0	6.0
Fine Motor Composite	3.0	6.0
Total Battery Composite	2.0	4.0
Short Form	3.0	6.0

[a]Median values from all possible scores

Figure 3.7 presents the *Bruininks-Oseretsky Test* scores plotted on the MSI profile with ±2 standard errors of measurement around the individual's score values of our example.

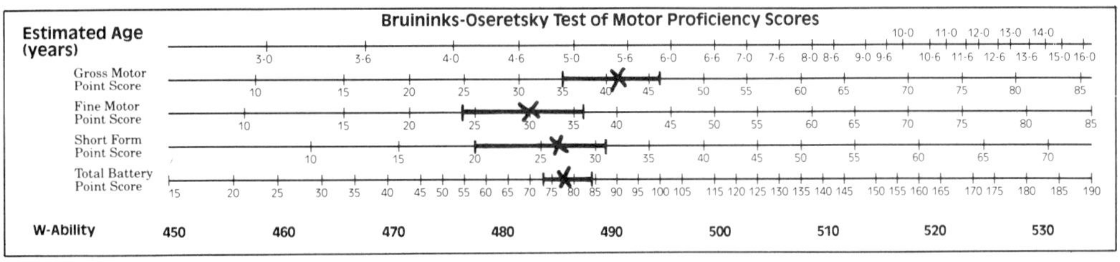

Figure 3.7. *Bruininks-Oseretsky Test* scores, showing standard errors of measurement, in the MSI profile

Step 4: Estimate performance on MSI skill items from *Bruininks-Oseretsky Test* scores. This step provides the user with several options. Ordinarily, the user will select only one *Bruininks-Oseretsky Test* score to predict performance on MSI skill items. Although the profile permits use of all four *Bruininks-Oseretsky Test* scores, it is recommended that users use the Gross and Fine Motor composite scores listed in Table 3.2 in projecting performance ranges for the modules on the MSI. The Total Battery or Short Form scores, while very useful, would be considered somewhat less desirable, since they are based on performance derived from a much broader, more heterogeneous range of tasks.

Table 3.2
Recommended *Bruininks-Oseretsky Test*
Scores
Used to Predict MSI Performance

MSI Module	Recommended B-O Scores
Body Management	Gross Motor Composite
Locomotor	Gross Motor Composite
Body Fitness	Gross Motor Composite
Object Movement	Gross Motor Composite
Fine Motor	Fine Motor Composite

Returning to Figure 3.7, the estimated performances on MSI Body Management items are found by drawing or visualizing two vertical lines from the ±2 standard errors of measurement points for the Gross Motor Composite score. This range of estimated performance on the MSI Body Management skill items is illustrated in Figure 3.8.

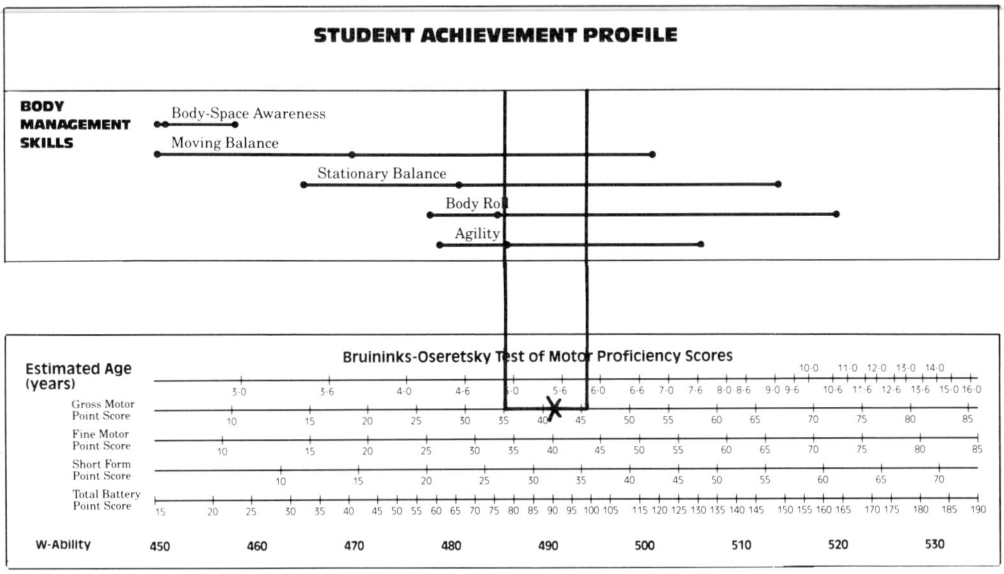

Figure 3.8. Expected range of performance on MSI body management items based on the *Bruininks-Oseretsky Test* Gross Motor Composite score

This procedure of marking the range of expected performances on the MSI items from the *Bruininks-Oseretsky Test* Gross Motor and Fine Motor Composite scores is shown completed for the remaining modules in Figure 3.9. Please note that the *Bruininks-Oseretsky* Fine Motor Battery scores were used to establish the ranges for the MSI Fine Motor Module. The same procedural steps may be followed using the Short Form and Total Battery scores.

The illustrations of the assessment strategy thus far have assumed that the *Bruininks-Oseretsky Test* was administered initially to students in the program. It is possible to bypass this step and directly administer the MSI. In this case, the user would administer the MSI, following the instructions in Appendix A, mark the student's performance in the MSI Record Booklet, and then plot the student's actual performances on the profile on the back of the record booklet. For example, the student may have the scores illustrated in Figure 3.10 for the locomotor items on the MSI.

These scores are then plotted on the back of the MSI Record Booklet with an (X) denoting the highest level achieved for each item, as shown in Figure 3.11. This score plotting displays a student's pattern of performance across items and modules of the MSI. The profile also provides general estimated ages for items of the MSI. These estimates should not be interpreted as age equivalent scores.

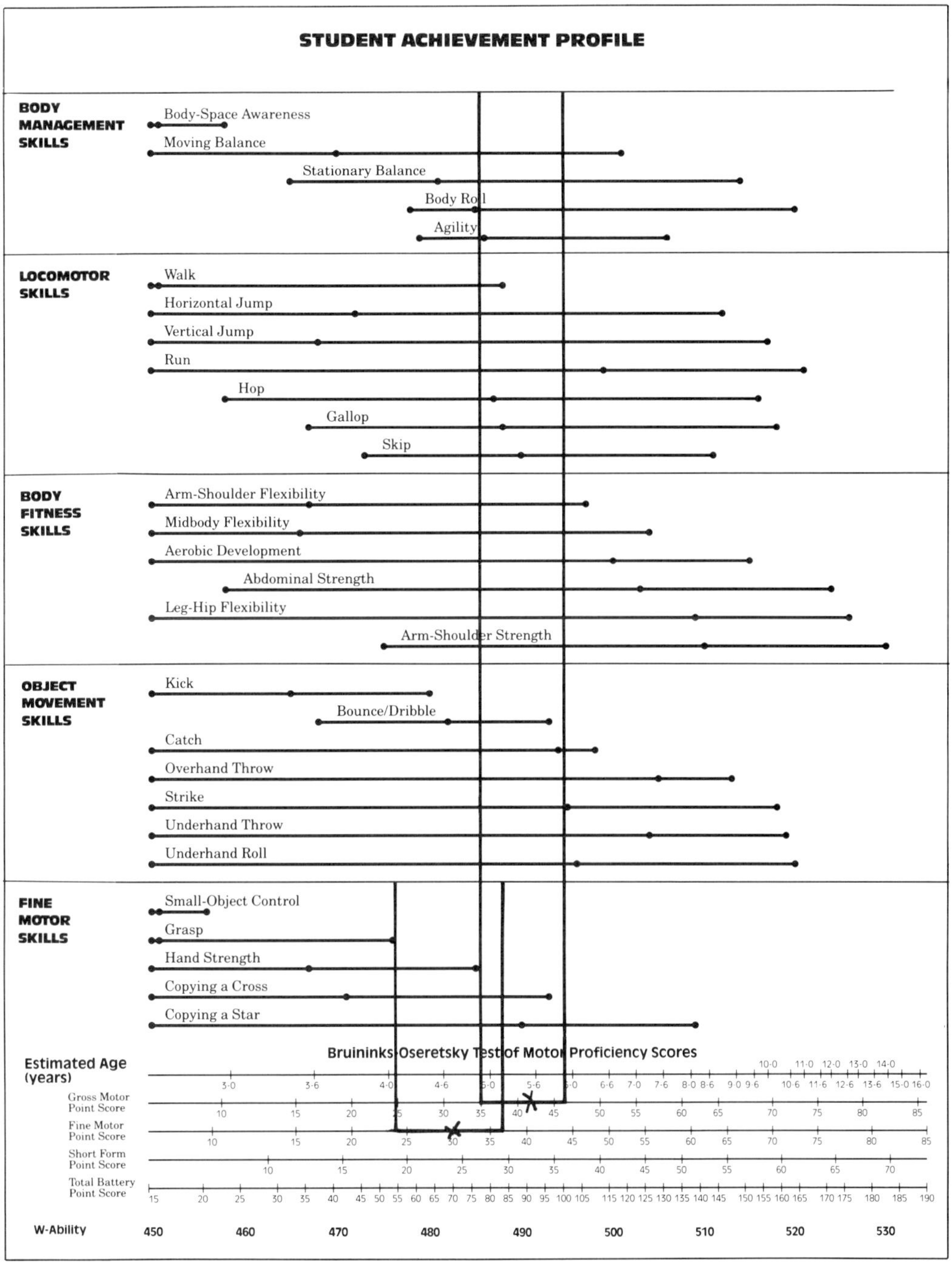

Figure 3.9. Expected range of performance on MSI items based on *Bruininks-Oseretsky Test* Gross Motor Composite and Fine Motor Composite scores

Locomotor Skills

Walk		Score + or −
RUDIMENTARY	Walking with a wide base of support	+
FUNCTIONAL	Walking flat-footed	+
*MATURE	Walking smoothly	+

Horizontal Jump		
RUDIMENTARY	Jumping upward with uneven landing	+
FUNCTIONAL	Jumping forward with arms and legs uncoordinated	+
*MATURE	Jumping forward with arms and legs coordinated	−

Vertical Jump		
RUDIMENTARY	Jumping slightly upward and forward with arms at sides	+
FUNCTIONAL	Crouching and jumping with arms above head	−
*MATURE	Jumping with one arm extended upward	−

Run		
RUDIMENTARY	Running flat-footed with wide base of support	+
FUNCTIONAL	Running with arm opposition and short strides	−
*MATURE	Running with arm opposition and long strides	−

Hop		
RUDIMENTARY	Hopping with slight knee bend, minimal balance	+
FUNCTIONAL	Hopping with full knee bend, exaggerated arm swing	+
*MATURE	Hopping with full knee bend, coordinated arm movements	−

Gallop		
RUDIMENTARY	Galloping flat-footed	+
FUNCTIONAL	Galloping with rocking motion	−
*MATURE	Galloping with long strides	−

Skip		
RUDIMENTARY	Skipping stiffly in a step-hop pattern	−
FUNCTIONAL	Skipping with exaggerated, airborne hop	−
*MATURE	Skipping rhythmically	−

3

Figure 3.10. Sample module section from MSI Record Booklet

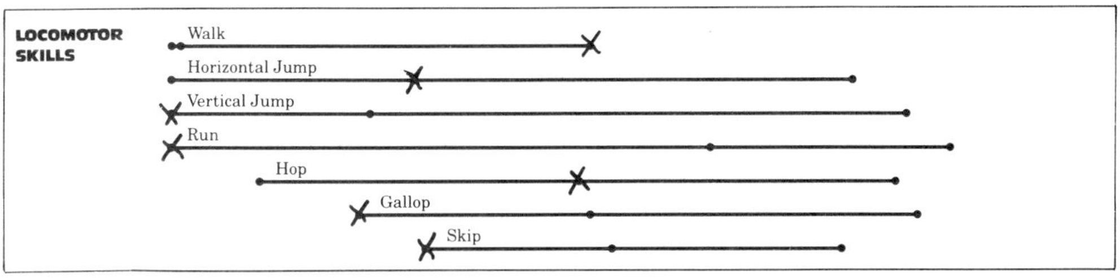

Figure 3.11. Locomotor profile from MSI Record Booklet

Step 5: Select teaching activities. Selecting activities for instruction is best done by evaluating the assessment results and comparing them with overall program goals, and more specifically, goals that seem most desirable for providing needed practice for the greatest number of students.

The MSI profile is useful in identifying the modules and specific motor skills in which the student most needs instruction. By plotting and reviewing the results, teachers can identify areas in which students need further training.

Selecting instructional activities requires judgment and decision making. *Body Skills* is designed to be flexible to meet instructional priorities. Activity selection should be based upon a knowledge of individuals in a group, their level of interest in the activities, and the program goals.

Developing Group and Individual Educational Plans

The previous section describes assessment strategies to be used before selecting and teaching the *Body Skills* activities. These steps followed the assessment-intervention strategies presented in Figure 3.1. The assessment-intervention strategies can be used to organize group instruction or to develop individualized educational plans (IEPs) according to state and federal regulations.

Typically, individualized educational plans include the following components:

- Assessment of present level of performance
- Statement of annual goals
- Statement of objectives and criteria for attainment
- Reason for type of educational program
- Types of services needed, amount of time, duration, and their location
- Plan and schedule for periodic review and evaluation

The design of the *Body Skills* curriculum and materials makes it relatively easy to design explicit individual educational plans.

The *Body Skills* program includes a number of useful instructional planning aids. The MSI profile on the back of the MSI Record Booklet will provide an overview of the student's developmental level on the skills assessed by the MSI. The Class Record Forms, included with the *Body Skills* blackline masters, can be used to record students' levels of performance for each module. Figure 3.12 presents a completed record form for the Locomotor Module for a group of five students in an adaptive physical education program. The MSI levels recorded on the Class Record Form present the performance levels at different times for students in a group. For Roland, walking was performed at a functional level during the first evaluation (9/20). He performed the walking skill items at a mature level in the next evaluation (10/4). Examination of performances on the MSI for this group of students indicates that they are mostly functioning at early developmental levels on these tasks.

LOCOMOTOR SKILLS
Class Record Form

Class *Mr. Skaar* Period *3*

Instructions: Record the date for each evaluation. For each student, record R for *rudimentary* performance, an F for *functional* performance, or an M for *mature* performance.

Students' Names / Skill:	Crawl			Walk			Horizontal Jump			Vertical Jump			Run			Hop			Gallop			Skip		
Date:				9/20	10/4	11/6	10/15	1/10	4/6	11/6	1/30	3/10	10/5	11/20	1/5	11/20	2/5	4/20	1/5	4/11	5/20	4/10	4/30	5/10
Roland O'Leary				F	M	M	R	R	F	R	R	R	F	M	M	R	F	M	F	F	M	R	R	F
Rita Teves				M	M	M	F	M	M	R	F	M	M	M	M	R	F	M	M	M	M	F	M	M
Sara Steck				R	R	F	R	R	F	R	R	R	R	R	R	R	R	R	R	F	F	R	R	R
Joshua Nelson				R	F	F	R	R	R	R	R	R	R	R	F	R	R	R	R	F	F	R	R	R
Brian Green				F	F	M	F	F	M	F	F	F	F	F	M	R	R	F	F	F	M	R	F	F

Figure 3.12. Completed Class Record Form for locomotor skills

The Individualized Educational Planning (IEP) Form is provided to assist teachers in selecting instructional activities for individual students. This form is also provided on a blackline master that can be duplicated. The IEP form may be used after the MSI results have been reviewed (see Figure 3.13). It provides a place to list IEP goals and objectives for teaching motor skills, the *Body Skills* activities to be taught, and the MSI items to be administered for evaluation of instruction.

INDIVIDUAL EDUCATIONAL PLANNING FORM

Name: Jackie Washington Grade: K Birthdate: 9/26/82

IEP Meeting Date: 11/17/88 Dates for reviewing plan: 3/17/89

Case Manager: Tony Scarpelli Classroom Teacher: Susan Wolf

GOALS	OBJECTIVES	ACTIVITIES	EVALUATION PLAN
To develope and improve body management skills	Given a two-inch tape line ten feet long, demonstration, and verbal direction, the student will walk heel to toe down the line with hands on hips demonstrating a mature pattern two out of three times	Moving Balance Activities 1. Connections 2. Safari 3. Beanbag Tag 4 Walk the Line 5. Canyon Cross 6. Copy Cats	Administer MSI Body Management items
To develope and improve locomotor skills	Given a 20-foot distance, demonstration, and verbal direction, the student will demonstrate a mature galloping pattern two out of three times	Gallop Activities 1. Gallop-Go-Round 2. Horse Pairs 3. Wild and Tame Horses 4 Gallop Away 5. O.K. Corral 6. Caravans	Administer MSI Locomotor items
To develope and improve object movement skills	Given a stationary 8-to-10-inch kicking ball, a target, verbal direction, and demonstration, the student will kick the ball using a mature kicking pattern two out of three times	Kick Activities 1. Kick Off 2 Call and Kick 3 Through the Mountains 4 Circle Kick 5 Kick and Trade 6. Line Kick 7. Kick It Over 8. Guard Ball	Administer MSI Object Movement items

Figure 3.13. Completed Individual Educational Planning Form

Following the assessment of motor skills, the teacher must select skill areas that students most need to develop. This task clearly requires some judgment, based upon an overall assessment of the learner's abilities and skills. When the skill areas are identified, parts of the individualized plan can be detailed. The primary focus then changes to listing the goals, objectives, and criteria for their attainment, the instructional activities, and a plan for periodic review and evaluation.

Step 1: Establish goals. The *Body Skills* curriculum provides a convenient means for identifying instructional goals. Let's assume that the teacher decides to work on skills in the Body Management, Locomotor, and Object Movement

Modules. These broad goals can be written into the student's individual educational plan (see Figure 3.13):

To develop and improve body management skills.
To develop and improve locomotor skills.
To develop and improve object movement skills.

Step 2: Identify objectives. The materials are designed for easy formulation of specific instructional objectives. The teacher begins by selecting particular skill areas. Assume that the teacher decides to work on moving balance skills (Body Management Module), on galloping (Locomotor Module), and kicking (Object Movement Module). The objectives and the criteria for their achievement may be taken and written into the IEP form directly from the MSI items, which are also objectives in the *Body Skills* program. Based on school district requirements, objectives may be written simply, as in the *Body Skills* activities, or as behavioral objectives; for example:

1. *Given a two-inch tape line ten feet long, demonstration, and verbal direction, the student will walk heel-to-toe down the line with hands held on hips demonstrating a mature pattern two out of three times (all steps placed on the line in a heel-to-toe pattern).*
2. *Given a 20-foot distance, demonstration, and verbal direction, the student will demonstrate a mature galloping pattern two out of three times (steps with same foot as lead leg with arm-leg opposition).*
3. *Given a stationary eight-to ten-inch kicking ball, a target, verbal direction, and demonstration, the student will kick the ball using a mature kicking pattern two out of three times (steps toward ball with arm-leg opposition, follows through with legs straight).*

Step 3: Select teaching activities. In this step, the teaching activities are simply listed by reference number and title, as shown in Figure 3.13.

Step 4: Schedule periodic evaluation. The final step is to reference the MSI items to assess the student's progress and to plan a schedule for administering them (see Figure 3.13).

The next section provides an actual completed case illustration of the assessment, curriculum planning, intervention, and evaluation of the concepts discussed in this chapter.

A Case Study

This section presents a case study to illustrate implementation of the assessment-intervention process of the *Body Skills* program. The following case study is an example of the manner in which the *Bruininks-Oseretsky Test* and the MSI data (Option 3; see Figure 3.1) can be used for decision-making purposes.

Background Information. Miguel is four-years, nine-months old, of average height, slender build, and in good health. He attends preschool three hours a day during the week. At a recent child study team meeting, his preschool teacher requested that Miguel be assessed by the adaptive physical education specialist.

She noted that Miguel appeared clumsy, exhibited poor motor skills, and showed little interest in physical activities.

Assessment Data. *Bruininks-Oseretsky Test Results.* The full scale test was administered in two 30-minute segments. Miguel's performance on the Gross Motor Subtests ranged from below that of an average four-year-two-month-old in Running Speed and Agility and Bilateral Coordination to that of an average four-year-eight-month-old in Balance. His performance is below that of his actual chronological age, and he performed Gross Motor Skills equal to or better than only 18 percent of his chronological age peers in the norming sample. Results of Miguel's test performance are presented in Figure 3.14.

Miguel's performance on the Fine Motor Subtests ranged from below that of an average four-year-two-month-old in Response Speed to a five-year-eight-month-old in Visual-Motor Control. His performance in Upper-Limb Speed and Dexterity was at age-level. Miguel performed fine motor skills equal to or better than 58 percent of his chronological peers in the norming sample.

The Battery Composite score indicates that Miguel is functioning at the 38th percentile, or slightly below his chronological age in general motor ability. The Gross Motor Composite score is below age-level while he is performing at age-level in fine motor skills. The specific areas of motor deficit are Running Speed and Agility, Bilateral Coordination, and Response Speed.

At this point, the teacher could proceed to estimate Miguel's performance on skills in the *Body Skills* curriculum by plotting the *Bruininks-Oseretsky Test* scores on the MSI profile. These scores could then be used to predict Miguel's likely performance on the MSI skill items. The teacher could also administer the MSI along with the *Bruininks-Oseretsky Test*, or simply administer the MSI.

MSI Results. The entire five modules of the inventory were administered in one 30-minute session. Results of administering the MSI are presented in Figure 3.15. In Body Management, Miguel performed at or very close to the expected range of performance for his age in stationary balance, body rolling, and agility. However, in moving balance and body-space awareness, Miguel performed at a rudimentary level. He responded inconsistently in his ability to move his body in different directions in space and had difficulty in balancing while moving. In Locomotor Skills, Miguel performed hopping, galloping, and skipping skills at a rudimentary level. The horizontal jumping, vertical jumping, and running skills were performed at a functional level, indicating that most of the movements of the skill were performed but were not smoothly integrated. In Object Movement Skills, Miguel functioned at the rudimentary level. He demonstrated parts of the skill, but failed to integrate all movements in a coordinated manner. Miguel performed quite well on the Body Fitness items. All skills in flexibility were performed at the mature level and tasks involving strength were performed at a functional level. Consistent with the results of the *Bruininks-Oseretsky Test*, Miguel did very well in Fine Motor Skills, performing at the mature level. The MSI scores indicate that Miguel is functioning at a rudimentary level in Locomotor, Object Movement, and some Body Management skills, at the functional or mature level in Body Fitness, and at a mature level in Fine Motor skills.

BRUININKS-OSERETSKY TEST OF MOTOR PROFICIENCY / Robert H. Bruininks, Ph.D.

INDIVIDUAL RECORD FORM

COMPLETE BATTERY AND SHORT FORM

NAME *Miguel Arroyo* SEX: Boy ☒ Girl ☐ GRADE *Presch.*

SCHOOL/AGENCY *Sunnyside* CITY *Brownville* STATE *Iowa*

EXAMINER *S. Vetruta* REFERRED BY *Keelor*

PURPOSE OF TESTING *poor motor skills*

Arm Preference: *(circle one)*

RIGHT LEFT MIXED

Leg Preference: *(circle one)*

RIGHT LEFT MIXED

	Year	Month	Day
Date Tested	88	11	25
Date of Birth	84	2	14
Chronological Age	4	9	

Complete Battery:

SUBTEST	POINT SCORE Maximum	POINT SCORE Subject's	STANDARD SCORE Test (Table 23)	STANDARD SCORE Composite (Table 24)	PERCENTILE RANK (Table 25)	STANINE (Table 25)	OTHER
GROSS MOTOR SUBTESTS:							
1. Running Speed and Agility	15	0	6				-4-2
2. Balance	32	14	16				4-8
3. Bilateral Coordination	20	1	11				-4-2
4. Strength	42	4	14				4-3
GROSS MOTOR COMPOSITE		(19)	*47 SUM	41	18	3	4-2
5. Upper-Limb Coordination	21	(6)	*18				4-11
FINE MOTOR SUBTESTS:							
6. Response Speed	17	0	9				-4-2
7. Visual-Motor Control	24	11	23				5-8
8. Upper-Limb Speed and Dexterity	72	16	15				4-8
FINE MOTOR COMPOSITE		(27)	*47 SUM	52	58	5	4-8
BATTERY COMPOSITE		(52)	*112 SUM	47	38	4	4-5

*To obtain Battery Composite: Add Gross Motor Composite, Subtest 5 Standard Score, and Fine Motor Composite. Check result by adding Standard Scores on Subtests 1-8.

Short Form:

	POINT SCORE Maximum	POINT SCORE Subject's	STANDARD SCORE (Table 27)	PERCENTILE RANK (Table 27)	STANINE (Table 27)
SHORT FORM	98				

Figure 3.14. *Bruininks-Oseretsky Test* Individual Record Form for Miguel Arroyo

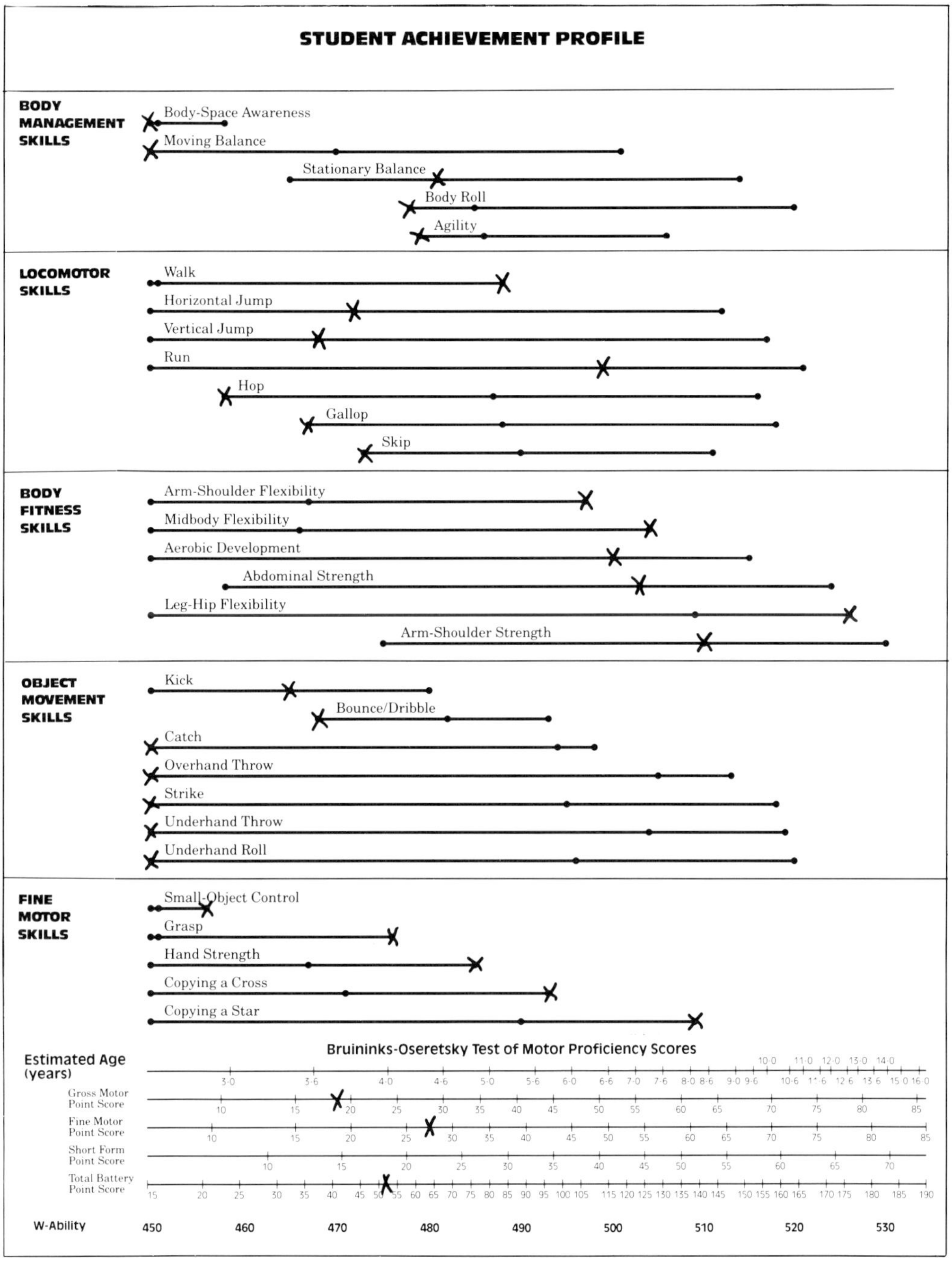

Figure 3.15. MSI Student Achievement Profile for Miguel Arroyo

Recommendations: Based on the *Bruininks-Oseretsky Test*, Miguel is functioning below age-level in gross motor skills, while his fine motor skills are at, or in some cases above, his chronological age level. Intervention is recommended with a focus on locomotor skills (running, hopping, galloping, skipping), object movement skills (kicking, catching, striking, throwing), and on some body management skills (body-space awareness, moving balance). *Body Skills* activities focusing on body management, locomotor skills, and object movement skills would be appropriate to address Miguel's individual needs. Miguel's reluctance to join in physical activity is of some concern; therefore, it is important that Miguel experience success in physical education activities. A reassessment of Miguel's gross motor skills is recommended in six months.

Summary of Assessment-Intervention Steps

Step 1: Administer the MSI and/or the *Bruininks-Oseretsky Test.*
Step 2: Translate results of performance into MSI profile.
Step 3: Select objectives and plan activities for instruction based on performance results.
Step 4: Implement instructional activities.
Step 5: Evaluate progress of students and select activities.

Evaluation

The final step in the program model for the *Body Skills* curriculum is evaluation of student progress and program goals. However, evaluation should not be considered a "last" step, but a key step in making decisions about further assessment and teaching. Evaluation involves determining the degree to which the goals and objectives of the program have been met. With the current emphasis in education on accountability, evaluation has become a crucial component of quality programs and is necessary for determining the success and effectiveness of implementing a program. This section presents suggestions for evaluating student outcomes and overall program effectiveness.

Student Evaluation

The heart of evaluation in education programs is concerned with answering the question: *What and how much did students achieve?* The initial assessment conducted with the students becomes the baseline of performance against which later evaluation is measured.

When assessment is an ongoing, periodic process, student evaluation consists of recording of performance levels following instruction. The levels of performance recorded during the school year can be presented in a profile showing growth in motor skill development. Figure 3.16 presents an example of recording results from curriculum-imbedded assessment for a single student using the Locomotor items on the MSI.

The same recording process can be followed to record the progress of an entire class using the Class Record Form. The Class Record Form for each of the *Body Skills* modules can be used to record class performance periodically throughout the school year. By examining growth in skill acquisition from the first recording to the last, the teacher can easily report the extent of student achievement that occurred during the program. Figure 3.17 presents an example of using the Class Record Form to record progress in achievement for a group or entire class.

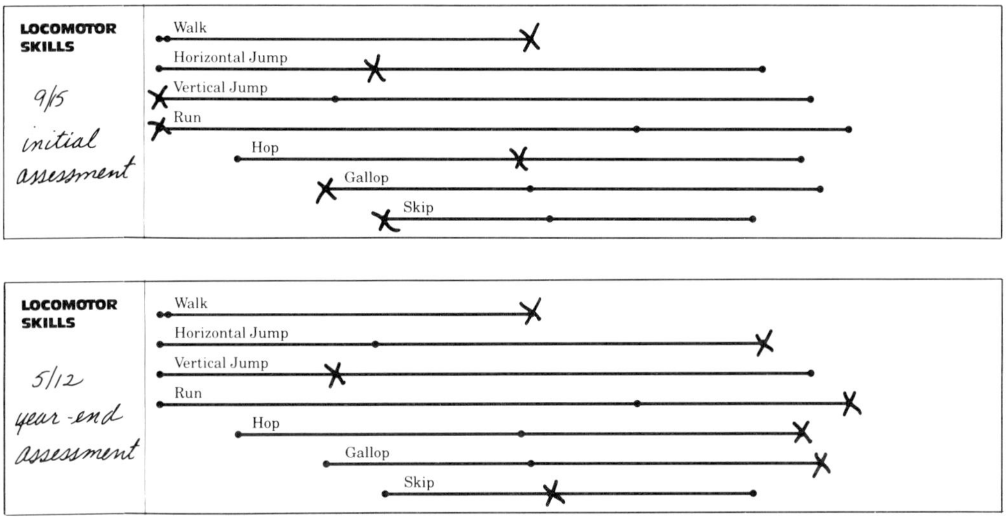

Figure 3.16. MSI profile showing student's performance on locomotor skills before and after instruction

If pretesting was conducted at the beginning of the program, similar posttesting should be conducted as a basis for measuring progress. If the *Bruininks-Oseretsky Test* was administered at the beginning of the program, it can be readministered at the end of the program. This test, as a measure of ability, is generally administered once or twice in a single school year. The MSI or its components can be administered more often, as a pretest, as an assessment throughout the year, and as a posttest measure. If both the *Bruininks-Oseretsky Test* and the MSI are administered, the profile on the last page of the MSI Record Booklet can be used to record results of both pretest and posttest administrations. The results of the second administration can be transferred to the MSI profile of the initial administration by using different colors to mark the profile (see Figure 3.18). This procedure graphically shows the motor skill progress of individual students throughout the school year on the MSI profile.

The Individual Skill Checklist may be used to record periodic assessments of each skill to show the progress of a particular student on any or all skills. Figure 3.19 demonstrates how the Individual Skill Checklist is used to show one student's progress.

While these forms are useful for displaying student achievement data, the importance of evaluation goes a step further. After assessing student progress, the next step is to measure growth on objectives specified in the program plan. Once students have established an achievement record, the degree to which objectives were met can be determined. For example, if the goal was to improve locomotor skills, and one of the objectives was to develop skill in hopping, a student's achievement in hopping should be evaluated by comparing the student's

BODY FITNESS SKILLS
Class Record Form

Class *Mrs. Langer* Period *3*

Instructions: Record the date for each evaluation. For each student, record R for *rudimentary* performance, an F for *functional* performance, or an M for *mature* performance.

Students' Names / **Skill:**	Arm-Shoulder Flexibility				Midbody Flexibility				Aerobic Development				Abdominal Strength				Leg-Hip Flexibility				Arm-Shoulder Strength			
Date:	9/15	11/15	1/15	3/7	9/15	11/15	1/15	3/7	9/15	11/15	1/15	3/7	9/15	11/15	1/15	3/7	9/15	11/15	1/15	3/7	9/15	11/15	1/15	3/7
Sara Chen	M	M	M	M	M	M	M	M	F	F	M	M	F	F	M	M	F	F	F	M	F	F	M	M
Leah Kuzma	F	F	M	M	F	M	M	M	R	R	F	F	R	R	F	F	R	F	F	F	R	R	R	R
David Cohen	M	M	M	M	M	M	M	M	M	M	M	M	F	M	M	M	F	M	M	M	F	M	M	M
Sam Sedak	M	M	M	M	F	M	M	M	F	F	M	M	F	F	M	M	F	F	M	M	F	F	M	M
Jason Lee	F	F	F	M	R	R	F	M	R	R	F	F	R	R	R	F	R	R	R	R	R	R	F	F
Anita Sanchez	M	M	M	M	M	M	M	M	M	M	M	M	M	M	M	M	M	M	M	M	M	M	M	M
Zachary Gomez	R	F	F	F	R	R	F	F	R	R	F	F	R	R	R	F	R	R	F	F	R	R	R	F
Marty Estrada	F	M	M	M	F	F	M	M	F	F	F	M	F	F	M	M	F	M	M	M	F	M	M	M
Mary Ann Yee	M	M	M	M	M	M	M	M	F	M	M	M	F	M	M	M	F	F	M	M	F	F	M	M
Jane Koch	R	F	F	F	R	R	R	F	R	R	F	F	R	R	F	F	R	R	F	F	R	R	R	F
William Brown	M	M	M	M	M	M	M	M	F	M	M	M	F	M	M	M	F	M	M	M	F	M	M	M
Mikki Estuesta	F	M	M	M	F	F	M	M	F	F	M	M	F	F	F	M	F	F	M	M	F	M	M	M
Leif Borgen	F	F	M	M	F	M	M	M	F	F	M	M	F	F	M	M	F	F	F	M	F	F	M	M
Laura Davey	M	M	M	M	M	M	M	M	M	M	M	M	F	M	M	M	M	M	M	M	F	M	M	M
Cassie Lunde	M	M	M	M	M	M	M	M	M	M	M	M	M	M	M	M	M	M	M	M	M	M	M	M

Figure 3.17. Class Record Form showing progress on body fitness skills

pretest level with later assessments using the MSI hopping items. If the student shows evidence of improvement, the objective has been met; if not, that is, if the student is still at the pretested level of skill performance, that particular objective was not met.

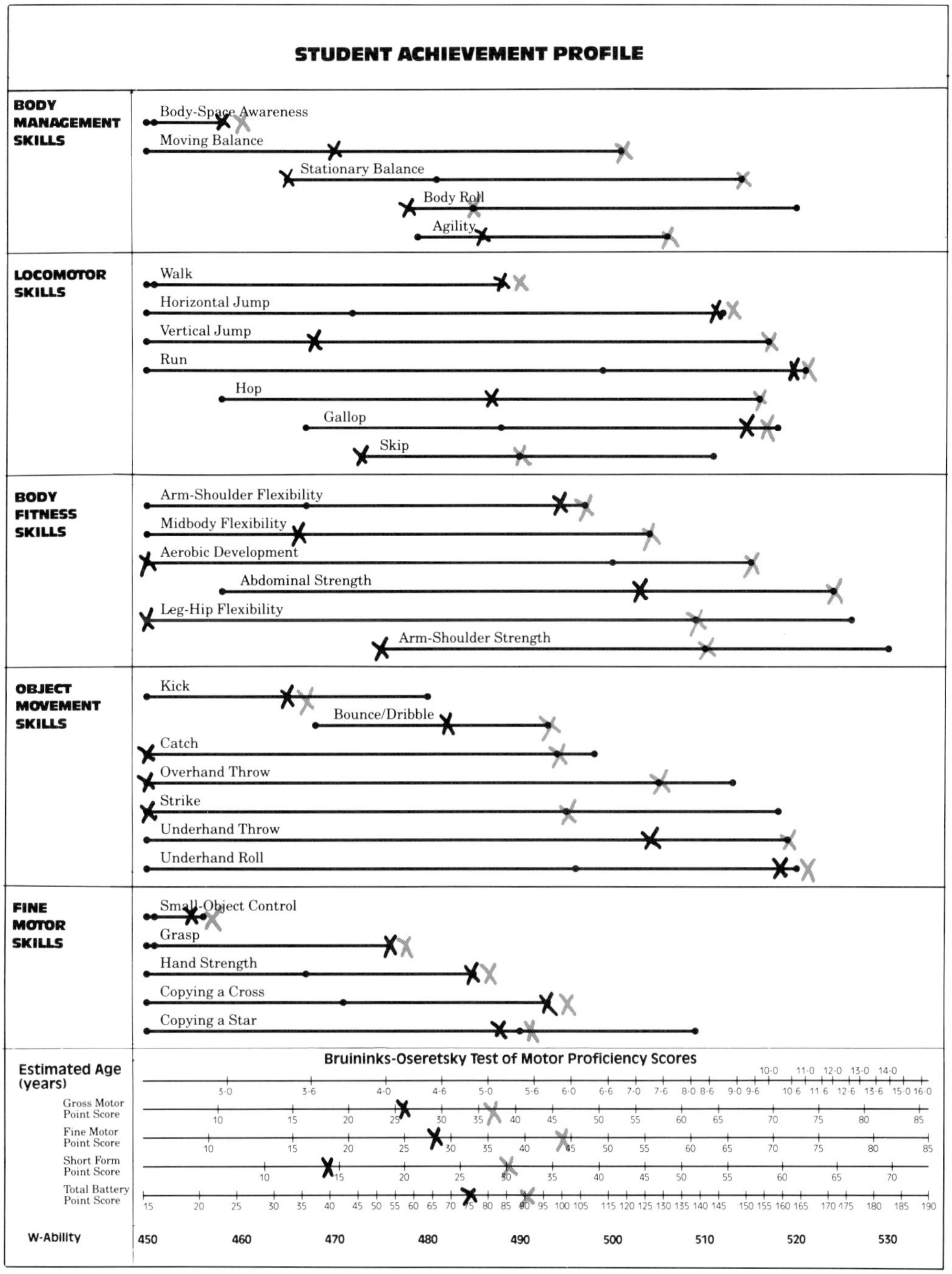

Figure 3.18. MSI profile showing pretest and posttest results from the *Bruininks-Oseretsky Test* and the MSI

INDIVIDUAL SKILL CHECKLIST

Name Leah Kocina Class Mrs. Erhardt

Period 1:45-2:15 MWF Grade 1 Birthdate 7-3-82

Instructions: Record the date for each evaluation. For each skill, record an R for *rudimentary* performance, an F for *functional* performance, or an M for *mature* performance.

Date:	9/15	1/15	5/1		
Body Management					
Body-Space Awareness	M	M	M		
Moving Balance	F	F	M		
Stationary Balance	M	M	M		
Body Roll	R	F	F		
Agility	F	M	M		
Locomotor					
Crawl	M	M	M		
Walk	M	M	M		
Horizontal Jump	M	M	M		
Vertical Jump	F	M	M		
Run	M	M	M		
Hop	M	M	M		
Gallop	M	M	M		
Skip	F	F	M		
Body Fitness					
Arm-Shoulder Flexibility	M	M	M		
Midbody Flexibility	M	M	M		
Aerobic Development	R	F	M		
Abdominal Strength	F	F	M		
Leg-Hip Flexibility	M	M	M		
Leg-Hip Strength	F	F	M		
Arm-Shoulder Strength	F	F	F		
Object Movement					
Kick	F	F	F		
Bounce	F	M	M		
Catch	F	F	M		
Overhand Throw	R	F	F		
Strike	R	F	F		
Underhand Throw	F	M	M		
Underhand Roll	M	M	M		
Fine Motor					
Small-Object Control	M		M		
Grasp	M		M		
Hand Strength	M		M		
Visual-Motor Control	M		M		

Figure 3.19. Individual Skill Checklist showing student's progress

When inadequate progress occurs on specific skill objectives, an examination should be conducted of the instructional process. Many reasons can be found for lack of student progress. Reasons of scheduling difficulty, lack of time spent on the objective, and frequent absences are just a few of the possible reasons. Perhaps hopping was not an appropriate objective for this particular student or a particular group of students. After examining the information, the program plan and objectives can be modified. If improving progress in hopping is still the objective, it should stay in the student's individualized plan, and some changes in teaching procedures should be considered.

A part of student evaluation that must not be neglected is evaluation of the student's attitude toward movement and physical activity, and toward her or his own physical fitness. The *Body Skills* activities are intended to enhance motor skill acquisition, and the activities were developed to provide enjoyable experiences as well as to develop self-confidence and cooperation among students. Teachers can note during the activities whether the students are demonstrating a high level of interest in an activity and should make a point of assessing student attitudes during the activities. An attitude questionnaire with a few simple questions can be administered at the beginning of the program, periodically during the program, or at the close of the program. A sample attitude questionnaire that can be used in conjunction with the *Body Skills* curriculum is presented in Figure 3.20. The questionnaire may be given to students in written form or verbally as a focus of discussion at the end of an activity or lesson.

Program Evaluation

The procedures used to conduct and record individual student evaluation can also be used to evaluate program effectiveness. The cumulative results of the class on the MSI, on the *Bruininks-Oseretsky Test*, progress on objectives in the program plan, and the results of an attitude questionnaire can be compiled and presented as a total program evaluation. However, even with all this information, it may be difficult to assess overall program effectiveness.

One method of assessing the program is to conduct a statistical test comparing the *Bruininks-Oseretsky Test* results, or other results, from pretest and posttest measures. However, this procedure usually requires a comparison group or standard, which may not be a possibility for most teachers.

A descriptive analysis of the results may be the most feasible way to evaluate the program. In this analysis, the teacher can report the following descriptive information:

1. The number of students in the class at the beginning and end of the program.
2. The names of assessment instruments administered with a report of the scores for all students in the class.
3. The amount of visible progress, using standardized scores, on the *Bruininks-Oseretsky Test*, or other measures, for all students.

Student's name ______________________

Date ____________ Class ______________________

Activity title ______________________

Did you have fun during this activity?

____

What do you like to do most during this class?

____

____

Do you like to play outdoors?

____

Do you like to play any sports? Which ones do you like?

____

What did you do best today?

____

____

Do you play or do exercises at home or in a recreation center?

____

____

What new things have you learned in this class?

____

____

Figure 3.20. Student attitude questionnaire

4. The amount of progress in MSI items, showing the numbers of students making improvements in skills from one developmental level to another, or the number of students achieving mature levels of performance.
5. The number of objectives achieved from the *Body Skills* curriculum in student individualized education plans.
6. Evidence of positive student attitudes in the class.
7. The actual amount of time spent teaching the curriculum as compared with the amount of time projected for teaching.

The results of a program evaluation are useful only to the extent that they influence subsequent decisions for modifying and improving educational programs. An effective program evaluation should reveal strengths and weaknesses in the program. These results should be considered and recommendations made for planning and modifying future instructional programs.

The *Body Skills* program provides a number of options for evaluating the needs of students, planning and selecting instructional activities, monitoring the results of teaching, and evaluating the outcomes of the teaching activities and suggested teaching strategies. By using these options as appropriate, an exciting program of activities can be provided that will enhance the physical, social, emotional, and overall development of children.

Chapter 4

Research and Development

The development of the *Body Skills* motor curriculum began as an effort to translate results from the *Bruininks-Oseretsky Test of Motor Proficiency* into meaningful instructional activities. This chapter reviews the development and field testing of the *Body Skills* program.

Rationale

It has been established and is widely accepted that instruction in motor skills is an essential component in the educational program for all children (Espenschade and Eckert 1967; Rarick 1961). Learning to move effectively within their home, school, and community environments is a vital part of children's development. However, not all children are readily able to move well. For children with developmental disabilities, motor development typically progresses at a slower rate (Bruininks 1974; Rarick 1961). Although the sequence of motor development may be similar for all children, the rate of learning frequently differs for those children with handicapping conditions.

Considerable interest has been shown for the inclusion of appropriate physical education and motor skills training in schools and preschool education programs. In recent years, an emphasis upon fitness, nutrition, and health has led to an explosion of exercise centers, books, and individual exercise activities. This increased consciousness of the benefits of sound exercise and good health is reflected in requirements for physical development activities in preschool, elementary and secondary schools, and postsecondary educational programs. Physical activity is now clearly recognized as a valued aspect of development for children that is necessary for physical health.

The benefits of physical activity are recognized as particularly important to the development of children and youth with disabilities. In 1975, with the passage of Public Law 94-142, children with handicaps were guaranteed an education that included appropriate physical education activities. The law states that such education must include the development of physical and motor fitness and fundamental motor skills and patterns, and skills in aquatics, dance, and individual and group games and sports. Physical education, the only curriculum area specifically defined in this mandate, received a new emphasis in schools. Regular and special education teachers, preschool educators, physical education teachers, adaptive physical education specialists, and other therapists were challenged with the task of developing motor instructional programs for learners with handicaps.

Physical activity and recreation programs for students with handicaps have been developed and expanded throughout the country. To meet the requirements of legal mandates, many school districts developed adaptive physical education programs and served the physical activity needs of students with handicaps through separate, but highly individualized, classes. To meet requirements outlined in the mandate to place learners with handicaps in least restrictive educational environments, educators have been increasingly challenged to provide individualized physical education instruction in regular education environments. The concept of mainstreaming students with handicaps received tremendous national attention as a result of Public Law 94-142. Physical education classes and movement activities became an area in which mainstreaming was most likely to occur. The adaptive physical education movement endeavored to ensure that each student received appropriate motor training activities designed to meet her or his unique needs whether in the mainstream setting or in largely separate classes. Consequently, requirements to serve learners with handicaps raised the dilemma for regular physical education personnel concerning the best ways to provide instruction in motor skills within regular physical education classes.

The increased emphasis on physical activity in schools and in society generally has not been matched by the development of sound educational procedures and materials. The absence of good materials and procedures is particularly apparent in early childhood, elementary schools, and educational programs that serve children and youth with disabilities. Physical education teachers, classroom teachers, special education personnel, and early childhood educators who are faced with the challenge of preparing plans to teach important motor skills have few available curriculum resources that meet conceptual and practical standards of sound teaching. In recent years, government agencies in many states have established curriculum guidelines for physical education programs. While state guidelines specify instructional objectives to be taught, and often time requirements at each grade level, the development of plans and resources are typically left to teachers. The *Body Skills* program was designed to meet this need by providing teachers with assessment tools and suggested teaching activities to develop the motor skills and patterns of movement of children between the ages of two and 12 years, both children with handicapping conditions and nonhandicapped children.

Procedural Model for Curriculum Development

The review of literature on motor training and an evaluation of current practices and materials resulted in the development of a systematic process for the development of the *Body Skills* program. Figure 4.1 presents the procedural steps used to develop the MSI and the curriculum materials. This model was based on elements of Stake's formative evaluation model in identifying the stages involved in achieving the goals and objectives of a project (Stake 1967) and assuring effective management of actions and resources used in developing the materials.

The procedures that followed in the development of the *Body Skills* program were also guided by Von Bertalanffy's systems approach toward curriculum development (Von Bertalanffy 1968). The systems approach to design and development offers a logical and orderly process for making curriculum decisions.

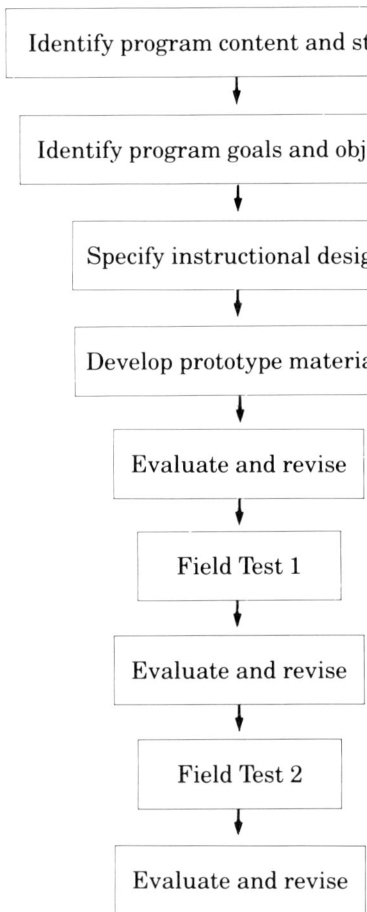

Figure 4.1. Procedural model followed for development of the *Body Skills* curriculum

Program Structure and Content

The conceptual framework of the *Body Skills* program, as an instructional system, is based on established principles and validated sequences of motor development in children. Based upon a thorough review of existing research studies, the instructional content was first organized into five broad motor domains:

Body Management
Locomotor
Body Fitness
Object Movement
Fine Motor

The motor areas were selected according to two criteria: (1) the identification of vital, functional skills in the psychomotor domain, as established by motor development experts, research studies, and reported observations of children's motor development; and (2) the selection of observable, measurable motor performance objectives, rather than underlying motor abilities. These general motor domains provided the preliminary conceptual design for the curriculum content. These motor domains were also linked conceptually to the *Bruininks-Oseretsky Test* (see Figure 1.3) so that following examination of test results for a student, a teacher would be able to readily determine which motor areas would constitute possible instructional goals to be incorporated into a lesson plan or an individual educational plan.

Following development of the conceptual design for the curriculum, criterion-referenced test items were then developed that could be used to evaluate the selection of activities, the placement of learners in the program, and the progress of learners during the period of training. These test items, linked conceptually to activities in the *Body Skills* curriculum, comprise the MSI and were also statistically equated to scores on the *Bruininks-Oseretsky Test*. (See Chapter 3 for a description of the assessment-intervention system.) Subsequently, through the use of the curriculum, the teacher would be able to select performance objectives with specific, appropriate instructional activities, each step in the process linked to the *Bruininks-Oseretsky Test* and the MSI to yield an efficient and integrated assessment, placement, and evaluation system.

Program Goals and Objectives

The five general motor domains or modules constituted the framework for generating instructional goals and more specific skill objectives. Chapter 1 presents an overview of the *Body Skills* curriculum and the skill areas that form the basic organizational framework for the curriculum (see Figure 1.1). It was planned that instructional objectives would be designed for every motor skill area. Within the curriculum itself, each of the motor skills was to be presented in an observable, measurable, and objective format to facilitate development of lesson plans and individual educational plans by teachers.

As the skill areas of the program were identified, available theoretical and research literature on each specific motor skill was studied in order to define its developmental sequence in normal children. One of the objectives in defining these developmental progressions was to present the development of each motor skill in a manner that would be easily understood by untrained, as well as trained, physical education, early childhood, and special education teachers and other educational personnel. Through carefully, operationally defined descriptions and clear illustrations, the basic stages of motor development of each skill were defined. These stages then became the basis for the evaluation criteria used for items in the MSI. The assessment was to provide a link to the instructional activities and was designed to emphasize the elements of mature levels of performance for each skill.

Following the identification of the modules and skills, the following goals and objectives were formulated to guide development of the specific materials. These goals and objectives reflect the developmental needs of children in movement exploration and physical activities and the practical needs of teachers. The curriculum goals provided criteria for designing the scope and structure of the curriculum. The curriculum objectives served to identify specific concepts, skills, and values that were considered essential. The overall purpose of the project was to develop a comprehensive and efficient assessment and intervention program that was based on established developmental principles of motor development in children. The following goals and objectives guided development of the *Body Skills* curriculum:

Curriculum Goals

1. To provide a motor instructional program appropriate for use with children from ages two to 12.
2. To provide a comprehensive program for instructing motor skills that are typical to all children.
3. To provide descriptions of the basic principles and sequences of motor skill development in children in typical physical activities.
4. To provide guidelines for the use of this curriculum in the program planning, intervention, and evaluation phases of instruction.
5. To provide procedures to assess developmental levels of basic motor skills.
6. To provide guidelines for the selection of motor skills in planning instructional activities.
7. To provide motor instructional activities that incorporate strategies appropriate for use with children with handicaps and nonhandicapped children.
8. To provide guidelines and efficient measurements for evaluating the results of instruction.
9. To provide motor activities for class, small group, and individual instructional settings.

Curriculum Objectives

1. To enhance proficiency of children and youth (ages two to 12) in functional gross motor and fine motor skills.
2. To facilitate transfer of motor skill learning to each child's social, academic, and home communities.
3. To promote development of positive self-images in children while moving in school, home, and community environments.
4. To encourage appropriate social behaviors in group motor activities.
5. To promote a functional vocabulary of motor concepts.
6. To promote functional self-help skills through movement tasks.

Designing the Curriculum

The principles and sequences of motor development based upon published research findings were taken into consideration in developing specifications for the *Body Skills* curriculum. The curriculum presents motor skills in a general developmental sequence. Later, after the results of the equating study, sequences were revised in accordance with findings that indicated developmental age markers. Details of the equating study are presented in Chapter 5. The following instructional conditions were also considered in specifying the instructional design and curriculum materials:

1. The content and the conceptual design were based upon available research regarding the development of motor skills in children.

2. The characteristics of the target populations for the curriculum were established for the developmental range of about two through 12 years.
3. The resources and situational factors in typical teaching environments were considered in designing all teaching activities.

Practical Considerations
This section describes the general considerations and specifications that were used in designing the *Body Skills* curriculum. In the development of *Body Skills*, the conditions under which the materials were most likely to be used were taken into consideration. Physical education teachers, early childhood teachers, elementary education teachers, special education teachers, and school therapists have limited amounts of preparation time and work with a wide variety of students. The *Body Skills* curriculum was designed to be flexible in order to meet the needs of a variety of situations. The activities provide specific instructions for implementing the teaching of motor skills and include a variety of ways each activity can be modified to increase its possible use in teaching situations. Sizes of activity areas and gymnasiums vary from school to school, and teachers have available to them different kinds of equipment. The space and equipment requirements for each activity were made as flexible as possible to meet the wide range of teacher settings and equipment. Special illustrations are included for each activity to guide the teacher in the general organization of learners and equipment. Materials required for each activity in the *Body Skills* program are typical physical education equipment items that are found in most schools.

Most physical education and motor activity programs are taught in a group or class setting. With the development of adapted physical education classes, some programs are taught in small groups or one-to-one. The *Body Skills* activities may be used with a large group of 15 to 30 students but may be easily adapted for small groups or for individual practice. *Body Skills* activities are designed for large group situations to reinforce the concept of mainstreaming children with disabilities into settings with nonhandicapped children. Guidelines for adapting activities for students with specific handicapping conditions are addressed on the skill folders and in Appendix B of this Manual.

Body Skills materials were designed to be portable and convenient for use in activity areas. Teachers who work as itinerant resource persons and teach at more than one school need materials that are portable and well-organized for easy use. The skill folders are clearly organized in a portable case, and the activity cards printed on durable cards. This format and organization make it convenient to use the program in nearly any setting.

Specifications
The instructional design underlying the *Body Skills* curriculum was intended to fill curricular needs in the fields of physical education, early childhood education, and special education. The instructional material was designed to serve children with handicaps and nonhandicapped children in a variety of situations. The curriculum meets the following specifications:

1. The activities provide practice in developmental sequences of motor skills for children, ages two to 12 years. All the motor skills are

described in three basic developmental levels (Rudimentary, Functional, Mature) to emphasize the progression of each skill toward a mastery level of performance.

2. The instructional activities allow practice at all levels in the developmental sequences of typical motor skills. The activities are designed to allow participation of children at all developmental levels of the particular motor skill (e.g., throwing).
3. A consistent teaching approach is presented for all skills in which the essential elements of the mature performance pattern is modeled and presented initially by the teacher even though all children may not be performing at that level.
4. The activities and instructions for teachers are written to emphasize validated principles of training in order to maximize efficiency and transfer of learning to everyday situations. The materials include suggestions and opportunities for reinforcement, repetition, and practice of motor skills.
5. The curriculum is divided into separate modules, one for each general motor area. Each module is clearly organized into its motor skill components that are cross-referenced to other related reinforcing motor activities within the curriculum.
6. The materials and activities, while presented in group settings, provide for individualization to accommodate the wide range of student characteristics and settings found in most teaching situations. Options for individualizing activities include: (a) instruction in a setting on a one-to-one student-teacher ratio; (b) grouping of students with consideration of their developmental levels, rates of learning, and learning styles; and (c) meeting the instructional needs of students with handicaps in the regular education settings to enhance their socialization with nonhandicapped peers.
7. The activities and materials are designed for ease, flexibility, and adaptability in school, clinical, home, or community settings.
8. The activities were designed as much as possible for use in group settings. The structure of most of the activities promotes interaction and socialization among students. Most activities are structured so that all students learn actively together.
9. The curriculum is adaptable for use with students of widely varying developmental and learning characteristics. The combination of the developmental approach to teaching motor skills with objective-based instruction makes it possible to individualize instruction for students with intellectual, emotional, sensory, or physical disabilities.
10. The activities include opportunities for reinforcing academic, creative, and daily living skills through the learning of motor skills.
11. The activities were designed to emphasize student-centered learning, by providing maximum time for movement and practice initiated by the student, with guidance provided by the teacher.
12. The directions for teachers use a variety of simple and direct auditory, visual, and physical cues in presenting activities.

13 The activities are structured to provide simple partner or group structures that minimize unhealthy competition among learners.
14. The activities require a minimal amount of equipment. The required equipment is typical to a variety of teaching situations and is relatively inexpensive, durable, and portable.
15. The equipment required for activities meets standards of safety, portability, and adaptability for students with handicaps.
16. The activity descriptions and procedures were written so as to be easily used by a variety of practitioners who may or may not have specific background or training in motor skill development, including classroom teachers, physical educators, early childhood educators, therapists, special education teachers, parents, and administrators.
17. The activities include a number of procedures for evaluation of the instructional activities. Procedures are included for monitoring students' progress toward attainment of developmental steps in the motor skill sequence using the MSI. Progress monitoring requires a minimal amount of time by the practitioner, and can be easily incorporated into an ongoing monitoring process.

Development of Prototype Materials

The translation of written specifications into an educational process and product involved several quality control steps. The abilities of talented developers and reviewers were employed throughout the process in order to make the materials and activities sensitive to the needs of serving children of a variety of ages and in a variety of settings. As the instructional materials were being written, they were subjected to formative evaluation, as recommended by evaluation experts (Cronbach 1963; Stake 1967). The formative evaluation process was a systematic, continuous process that guided the modification of materials using ongoing review of teachers and specialists at all stages of development. The goal during the evaluation process was to determine, in a systematic manner, the weaknesses and deficiencies within the instructional prototype, the application of the MSI, and the materials. Judging the success of the materials was based on the degree to which they met the goals, objectives, and specifications established for the *Body Skills* program and met the standards of external reviewers. Primary evaluation concerns were feasibility, appropriateness, and effectiveness in teaching fundamental motor skills and patterns. At the conclusion of the formative evaluation by practitioners, revisions were made and the prototype materials were prepared for use in two formal field tests.

First Field Test

After the internal evaluation was complete and the revision and preparation of the prototype materials were completed, a first field test of the materials was undertaken. The first field test was conducted as part of a larger study to conduct a formative evaluation of the curriculum materials. In this field test, 60 learning-disabled children, ages six to nine, in groups of one to three students, were randomly selected to receive instruction with the activities during a 12-week period. Two specially trained physical education teachers conducted the instruction in this formative evaluation of the curriculum. The teachers were presented the activities with minimal instructions or guidelines for their use. The teachers were asked to complete a rating form for each activity they taught. The rating form asked that each activity be evaluated using a five-point Likert rating scale with five indicating the highest rating according to appropriateness of: (1) form and content, (2) principles of learning, and (3) ease of implementing the activity. The rating form also included an area for recording comments and recommendations about the activity.

Raw scores from each teacher's review were tabulated and summed for each activity. Narrative review comments were not assigned numerical values and thus were not reflected in the empirical data, but were essential to evaluating and revising the materials.

A total of 34 representative activities were evaluated. In general, the formative evaluation of the motor curriculum activities indicated very high review scores (2007 out of a possible 2100, or 96 percent). The teachers agreed that the format and content of the activities were easy to read and understand. The evaluation further revealed that the activities adhered closely to principles of learning in terms of opportunities for practice, appropriateness, motivational qualities, clarity of directions, and safety. Implementation of the activities received the lowest ratings regarding how the activity worked with specific groups of students. It was apparent at this point in the development process that the strengths of the motor curriculum were in its format and content. Weaknesses indicated in the area of principles of learning appeared to be primarily editorial, with a few difficulties with the analyses of motor skills. Ratings from the formative evaluation also indicated selected problems with the implementation of the activities. This result seemed to be due to the fact that the reviewers rated the activity on how it worked with their particular groups, comprising one to three students, while frequently, the activity did not really allow easy application with groups of that size.

Based on this preliminary formative evaluation study, the following revisions and considerations were made in the curriculum design and materials:

1. The activities were revised to provide greater flexibility in use with large and small groups.
2. The skill sequence descriptions were revised to reflect findings from the literature on motor development more accurately.
3. Implementation of the activities was improved according to considerations that included: (a) suggestions to teachers for motivating students, (b) additional practice suggestions, and (c) additional instructional and environmental adaptations.

Common recommendations were incorporated into all activities, including those that were not evaluated. For example, the field-test results yielded insights into the time length of the activities, the availability of equipment, the appropriateness of directions, and their appeal to children.

The purpose of the field test was to evaluate the effectiveness of the initial motor curriculum activities. The field-test results were intended to assist in evaluating the feasibility, interest level, and the theoretical basis and practical aspects of the activities. Since the program under development was designed for use with physical education, early childhood, classroom, special education, and adaptive physical education teachers, further evaluation of the activities in a variety of settings was deemed essential to revising and improving the materials.

Second Field Test

After the recommendations and suggestions had been incorporated into the materials, a revised set of prototype materials was prepared for a second field test. These revised materials consisted of 206 curriculum activities. The materials were organized so that each participating teacher would be evaluating a total of 32 activities. The activities were organized into pairs, with each pair of activities constituting a complete lesson plan. Thus, there were 16 lesson plans for each teacher to implement and evaluate. Each teacher received a packet of 16 lesson plans, information explaining the materials, and a set of feedback forms. The materials were presented in a half-day training workshop by an experienced trainer. The workshop primarily covered procedural issues, with little guidance on how to implement the activities. In order to establish maximum external validity in evaluating the use of the materials in typical educational settings, it was considered vital that teachers implement the activities with little help or guidance, just as they would be expected to do in using a commercially available curriculum program for the first time.

Teachers were selected from California, Minnesota, and Texas to participate in the field test. A total of 46 teachers participated—24 from California, 13 from Minnesota, and 9 from Texas. Of the teacher sample, 19 were regular elementary physical education teachers, 18 were adaptive physical education teachers, and 9 were elementary classroom teachers. All 46 teachers returned feedback forms and comments on the lesson plans. A list of the field testers and the field-test sites is included in Appendix E.

For each implemented activity, each teacher was asked to complete a short survey-type feedback form about the activity. Figure 4.2 shows the evaluation form that was used for each activity. Teachers were encouraged to write their comments and suggestions directly on the lesson plans, to be compiled for further evaluative review. The evaluation forms and comments on the lesson plans were analyzed carefully. The first stage of the analysis included searching for suggestions or criticisms of the activities that were common to the basic format and structure of the activities. These elements were then taken into consideration and incorporated into the last revision of the activities. The second stage of the analysis involved a review of specific criticisms and suggestions for particular activities. Each activity was then revised to reflect these suggestions.

Skill ____________________ Activity ______________________________

Format and Content

_____ 1. The activity was easy to understand.

_____ 2. These elements were clear: set-up/equipment, organization of the activity, and directions to students.

3. Comments:

Principles of Learning

_____ 4. The activity provided practice of the motor skill.

_____ 5. The activity was appropriate for students regardless of handicapping condition.

_____ 6. The activity required social interaction and cooperation.

_____ 7. The activity was interesting and enjoyable to students.

_____ 8. Students were actively involved with the motor skill most (90%) of the class period.

9. Comments:

Implementation

_____ 10. This activity was successful with my students.

_____ 11. The given time frame was appropriate for this activity.

_____ 12. This activity was appropriate for the suggested age level.

_____ 13. The activity was straightforward and uncomplicated to use.

_____ 14. I would use this activity again.

Additional Comments and Recommendations:

Figure 4.2. Field-test evaluation form. Teachers evaluated each item using a five-point scale.

Chapter 5

Test Information and Equating Study

This chapter summarizes technical characteristics of the *Bruininks-Oseretsky Test of Motor Proficiency*, the equating study procedures linking the *Bruininks-Oseretsky Test* and the MSI, and the technical characteristics of the MSI.

Technical Characteristics of the *Bruininks-Oseretsky Test*

The eight subtests of the *Bruininks-Oseretsky Test* are designed to assess important aspects of motor development. Four subtests measure gross motor skills, three measure fine motor skills, and one measures both gross and fine motor skills. The performance on each composite is expressed as a normalized standard score with a mean of 50 and a standard deviation of 10. To obtain the most comprehensive information, test users are encouraged to administer the Complete Battery. However, Subtests 1-4 can be used alone to obtain an index of gross motor proficiency, and Subtests 6-8 can be used alone to obtain an index of fine motor proficiency.

Results of the *Bruininks-Oseretsky Test* are useful to educators, clinicians, and researchers in evaluating individuals for a variety of purposes. Recommended uses of the tests are described below.

1. Making decisions about educational placement.
2. Assessing gross and fine motor skills.
3. Developing and evaluating motor training programs.
4. Screening for special purposes.
5. Assisting clinicians and researchers.

The *Examiner's Manual* for the *Bruininks-Oseretsky Test* includes detailed information on the test's development and technical characteristics (Bruininks 1978). The test was standardized on a sample of nearly 800 subjects from three different regions of the United States and one region of Canada. The sample was quite evenly divided between male and female subjects, and quite closely approximated to the 1970 U.S. census statistics on race and community size.

In the *Bruininks-Oseretsky Test Examiner's Manual*, several forms of validity were presented from the original research on the *Bruininks-Oseretsky Test*, and many investigators have conducted technical studies since its initial publication. The available data indicates a rather strong relationship between the various scores of the test and chronological age, significant differences between individuals with handicaps and nonhandicapped individuals, and a variety of factor structure studies indicate support for the conceptual organization of the scale. Several forms of reliability are also presented for the scale and indicate that the test has good test-retest reliability and acceptable levels of interrater agreement for items requiring some degree of judgment. The test is used extensively throughout the United States and other countries as an evaluation measure to identify students in need of special services, and to design and evaluate curriculum and teaching programs. The reader is advised to consult a number of more recently published reports on the test and the *Examiner's Manual* (Bruininks 1978).

Equating *Bruininks-Oseretsky Test* and MSI Score Levels

To accomplish the equating of the *Bruininks-Oseretsky* point scores to the MSI items, the combined item sets of the *Bruininks-Oseretsky Test* (243 items) and the MSI (99 items) were calibrated together using the Rasch Analysis program. The Rasch scaling model (Hambleton and Cook 1977; Lord 1980; Rasch 1960; Wright 1968; Wright and Stone 1979) is a single-parameter logistic test model used for analyzing item response data. Test development procedures using this model are gathering increasing interest because of certain inherent advantages derived from these statistical procedures. Early applications of Rasch's work has resulted primarily from the efforts of Benjamin Wright at the University of Chicago. His efforts have resulted in the development of computer programs to analyze test data based on the Rasch model. One of the more comprehensive sources of information on the Rasch model, *Best Test Design* (Wright and Stone 1979), includes a comprehensive description of the Rasch model along with suggested procedures for its application. A variety of tests have been developed using the Rasch scaling procedures (Bruininks, Woodcock, Weatherman and Hill 1985; Woodcock 1978). These statistical procedures were used to equate the scores of the *Bruininks-Oseretsky Test* to the items of the MSI, so that the scores and items of the two respective measures could be arranged along a common scale of difficulty. In all analyses on the *Bruininks-Oseretsky Test*, point scores were used for the following measures: Gross Motor, Fine Motor, Total Battery, and Short Form. All profiles used as part of the MSI assessment and the curriculum program use the *Bruininks-Oseretsky* point scores.

The equating research sample consisted of 281 subjects (142 females and 139 males) ranging in age from three to 16 years (see Table 5.1). The mean age of the subjects was 9.21 while the median age was 9.00 (standard deviation = 3.17). No subject was excluded from the Rasch calibration due to abnormal person-fit statistics. The subjects were nonhandicapped students attending public schools in the metropolitan area of Minneapolis-St. Paul, Minnesota. Since the purpose of these analyses was to simply equate the two measures on a common scale, not to produce normative reference scores, it was considered unnecessary to construct a sample to be representative of the U.S. school population. Twenty-seven items were discarded by the Rasch program because all subjects got them correct (6 *Bruininks-Oseretsky* items, 21 MSI items), and 6 items were discarded because no one got them correct (all 6 were *Bruininks-Oseretsky* items). This left 309 usable items for calibration.

Table 5.1
Equating Study Sample

Age	Male	Female	Total
3.0-3.11	3	5	8
4.0-4.11	7	5	12
5.0-5.11	15	14	29
6.0-6.11	11	19	30
7.0-7.11	13	12	25
8.0-8.11	24	16	40
9.0-9.11	14	14	28
10.0-10.11	21	14	35
11.0-11.11	10	8	18
12.0-12.11	5	6	11
13.0-13.11	5	11	16
14.0-14.11	6	7	13
15.0-15.11	5	11	16
Totals	139	142	281

Two types of output from the Rasch analysis were used in constructing the "equating grids" for the age scale, the *Bruininks-Oseretsky* point scores and the MSI item scores for each item calibrated. The computer program produces a corresponding W-difficulty score. The W-scale is an equal interval open-ended scale (in both directions) with the mean for the hypothetical population fixed at 500 (Woodcock 1978). In addition, for any subject of the calibrated item pool (e.g., *Bruininks-Oseretsky* Gross Motor Battery Scores), the program provides a table which relates raw scores on the Battery to corresponding W-Abilities and W-Errors of estimate. Item difficulties (W-difficulties) and person abilities (W-abilities) are measured on the same scale. The mean W-Ability for the calibration sample was 510.2 and the median was 512.2. The subjects ranged in ability from 452.4 to 543.2 with a standard deviation of 17.6 W-score points.

One other type of data appears on the test equating grids, the age anchor information. These data were obtained by regressing W-Ability scores for the sample on the ages of subjects measured in months. There is a nonlinear relationship between W-Ability and age over the age range spanned by the sample. This fact necessitated that a Box-Cox transformation and a Box-Tidewell transformation be applied to the ability scores and age scores, respectively, prior to proceeding with a linear regression. Ability scores were transformed to natural-log-of-ability scores and age scores were transformed to one-divided-by-the-square-root-of-age scores. The final model had an R^2 of 89.1 percent. A Pure Error Test for Lack of Fit was performed against the obtained regression model and the resulting p-value was found to be 0.28 (meaning the analysis had a good fit). This model was then used to compute a table relating attained age (in months) to predicted W-Ability scores. The data were examined for possible sex differences in the relationship between W-Ability and age, but no statistically significant difference was found in these comparisons.

Technical Characteristics of the MSI

The MSI is designed to provide a qualitative measure of an individual's development and attainment of fundamental motor skills and patterns. Content for the scale was developed to provide a direct link to activities of the *Body Skills* curriculum. Items for the MSI were constructed based upon an extensive review of research and theoretical literature on the development of motor skills among children and youth (Corbin 1973; Cratty 1979; Espenschade and Eckert 1980). Skills and abilities considered indicative of important motor patterns of early childhood to adolescence were organized into conceptual categories according to current usage in the practice and in the professional literature. This produced an initial scale of over 125 items for field testing. These items were field tested extensively over several months with samples of students with handicaps and nonhandicapped students to produce the final scale.

Reliability. Two forms of reliability are presented for MSI scores. Table 5.2 presents Kuder-Richardson 20 reliabilities for the item clusters of the MSI. These reliabilities are generally in the .80s except for Body Fitness and Fine Motor Skills. The Body Fitness coefficient was close to .80; the internal consistency reliability for Fine Motor Skills was .63. The lower reliability for the Fine Motor items is likely due to the small number and heterogeneous quality of items in this particular cluster. Moreover, many subjects in this sample achieved perfect scores in these items, which would be expected to artificially lower the size of the correlation coefficient.

Table 5.2
Kuder-Richardson 20 Reliabilities
for MSI Item Clusters
(N=281)

Module	No. of Items (usable)	KR 20
Body Management	13	.82
Locomotor	17	.86
Body Fitness	15	.77
Object Movement	29	.88
Fine Motor	8	.63

Table 5.3 presents interrater reliability statistics for the MSI module raw scores. These scores were collected by having a second evaluator observe and score the test during its administration. Most of these coefficients are in the .70 range or above except for the Fine Motor cluster. The older subjects achieved mostly perfect scores on the Fine Motor items, again producing artificially low reliability coefficients.

Table 5.3
Interrater Reliability Statistics
for MSI Module Raw Scores

Module	Younger (N=22)	Older (N=24)
Body Management	.78	.83
Locomotor	.78	.59
Body Fitness	.73	.72
Object Movement	.68	.74
Fine Motor[a]	.66	NA

[a]Older subjects (above 8.0) mostly achieved perfect scores.

These limited studies show a reasonably good reliability for the MSI scores. As a result of the extensive field testing with the MSI, further refinements have been made in the scoring procedures and criteria. It is expected that subsequent studies will show somewhat greater consistency, and with higher internal consistency reliabilities and a better agreement among independent raters.

Validity. Several forms of validity statistics are presented in this section for the MSI. Table 5.4 presents Pearson product correlations and correlation ratios between the MSI module scores and chronological age for the equating sample. The correlations range between .67 and .73 in this sample. Correlation ratios (ETA^2) were considerably higher in most cases than the squared correlation coefficients. In the final column of this table are F-ratios indicating that most of the relationships between MSI scores and chronological age departed significantly from linearity. The departures from linear relationships resulted mostly from the scores reaching varying levels of maturity prior to the onset of adolescence. Most of the skill areas assessed by the MSI appear to reach a ceiling at approximately 10 to 12 years of age.

Table 5.4
Correlations Between
MSI Module Scores and Age
(N=281)

Module	r	r^2	ETA^2	F
Body Management	.67	.44	.67	15.28*
Locomotor	.73	.53	.59	3.32*
Body Fitness	.69	.48	.51	1.51
Object Movement	.70	.49	.53	23.09*
Fine Motor	.67	.44	.63	11.81*

*$p<.05$.

Table 5.5 presents correlations between MSI module and *Bruininks-Oseretsky Test* scores for the equating sample. These correlation coefficients are relatively high, mostly in the .70 to .83 range. There seems to be a rather high correlation between the total module scores of the MSI and the batteries and aggregate scores of the *Bruininks-Oseretsky Test*. Those areas assessing gross motor skills seem to have a somewhat higher correlation with the *Bruininks-Oseretsky* Gross Motor Battery than with the Fine Motor Subtests. Likewise, the Fine Motor section of the MSI produces a relatively high correlation with the Fine Motor Subtests of the *Bruininks-Oseretsky Test*. Reasonably high correlations, in the .70s, are also produced between the *Bruininks-Oseretsky* Short Form and the MSI module scores.

Table 5.5
Correlation Between
MSI Modules and *Bruininks-Oseretsky Test* Scores
(N = 281)

	Bruininks-Oseretsky Test Scores			
MSI Modules	Gross Motor Composite	Fine Motor Composite	Total Battery	Short Form
Body Management	.82	.79	.83	.79
Locomotor	.82	.73	.79	.78
Body Fitness	.73	.67	.72	.71
Object Movement	.75	.70	.75	.76
Fine Motor	.79	.78	.80	.77

Table 5.6 presents intercorrelations among the MSI module scores. Most of these correlations were between .60 and .70.

Table 5.6
Intercorrelations Among
MSI Module Raw Scores

Module	Body Management	Locomotor	Body Fitness	Object Movement	Fine Motor
Body Management	1.00	.70	.65	.54	.74
Locomotor		1.00	.68	.63	.66
Body Fitness			1.00	.50	.57
Object Movement				1.00	.60
Fine Motor					1.00

The data presented here on the validity of the MSI items and item clusters seems reasonably encouraging. The MSI items and the module raw scores seem to produce a reasonably strong relationship with chronological age, measures of motor development using the *Bruininks-Oseretsky Test*, and moderate to reasonably high intercorrelations among the module raw scores.

Appendix A

Directions for Administering and Scoring the Motor Skills Inventory (MSI)

The Motor Skills Inventory (MSI) is individually administered. It assesses an individual's development of 29 fundamental motor skills and patterns of movement. Most motor skills are divided into three developmental level test items; there are a total of 86 items. Examiners should read the following general instructions and the items for each skill carefully before administering the inventory.

A student's performance on the MSI is recorded in the MSI Record Booklet. Before administering the inventory, fill out the student information on the front of the Record Booklet.

To save testing time on some skills, begin by administering the item marked with an asterisk (*). If the student passes the marked item, assign a passing score to all items for that skill preceding the marked item, and administer the items that follow. If the student fails the marked item, administer the preceding items for that skill. If there is not a marked item for a skill, begin with the first item and, if the student passes, administer all items for that skill. Carefully observe the individual's performance to ensure that all elements of the performance or all actions at a particular skill level are performed correctly before awarding credit for passing it.

The MSI assesses the student's best level of performance. If a student displays the highest (mature) level of performance on a task for the first trial, and you are confident that it could be repeated, simply score it at the mature level and move on to the next item.

Allow students three trials to pass a skill item. Record a plus (+) for pass and a minus (−) for fail. Stop administering an item when the student passes it, and assign a passing score to all easier items for that skill. If the student fails on all three trials, do not administer the remaining items for that skill. Instead, score fail (−) for the higher items and proceed to the next skill.

On completing administration of the MSI, transfer the results to the Student Achievement Profile on the back of the Record Booklet. If available, transfer the results from the *Bruininks-Oseretsky Test of Motor Proficiency* to the profile to plot the results from both tests.

The following sections present more detailed instructions for organization, administration and scoring of each skill. *The MSI primarily assesses the quality of an individual's performance in relationship to criteria that have been arranged in a developmental hierarchy. Correct scoring depends upon the examiner's observation and judgment in relationship to the scoring criteria.*

Body-Space Awareness

Description:
This item assesses awareness of body parts and the ability to move them in response to verbal directions.

Equipment:
- none

Set Up:
Subject stands facing the examiner, about six feet away.

Directions:
Demonstrate actions while giving verbal directions. Then repeat the directions without demonstrating. See directions for each skill level.

Trials:
Allow up to three trials for each skill level. If the student demonstrates the actions correctly before the third trial, move on to the next skill level.

Scoring:
Score pass (+) if the student completes all actions correctly at each level.

RUDIMENTARY: Identifying Body Parts
Give the following directions one at a time.

Touch your arm.
Touch your leg.
Touch your hand.
Touch your elbow.
Touch your head.
Touch your foot.
Touch your knee.

FUNCTIONAL: Moving Body in Place
Give the following directions one at a time.

Sit down on the (chair or floor).
Stand up.
Turn completely (all the way) around.
Reach your arm up, put your arm down.
Bend your legs, straighten your legs.

MATURE: Moving Body in Space
Give the following directions one at a time.

Move forward four steps, move backward four steps.
Move sideways this way four steps (indicate direction), **move sideways four steps the other way.**
Move sideways four steps to the right. Move sideways to the left. (Give credit if the student moves three or more steps in each direction.)

Moving Balance

Description:
This item assesses the ability to balance the body while moving.

Equipment:

- two-inch floor tape

Set Up:
Make a ten-foot-long tape line on the floor. The student stands at one end of the line; the examiner stands beside the line, near the midpoint, to observe the student's steps.

Directions:
Demonstrate the actions while giving verbal directions. Then repeat the directions without demonstrating.

Trials:
Allow up to three trials for each skill level. If the student demonstrates the actions correctly before the third trial, move on to the next skill level. See directions for each skill level.

Scoring:
See directions for each skill level.

RUDIMENTARY: Walking on a Ten-Foot Line with Hands on Hips

Say: **Place your hands on your hips and walk to me on the line. Do not step off the line.**

Scoring: Score pass (+) if some part of the student's foot touches the line with each step of the ten-foot distance.

FUNCTIONAL: Walking on a Ten-Foot Line Stepping Heel to Toe for at Least Half of the Steps

Say: **Place your hands on your hips. When you walk, touch the toe of your back foot to the heel of your front foot. Walk this way to the end of the line.**

Scoring: Score pass (+) if the student's feet touch the line with each step, and a minimum of one-half of the steps are in a heel-to-toe pattern.

*MATURE: Walking on a Ten-Foot Line Stepping Heel to Toe for Each Step

Say: **Place your hands on your hips when you walk, touch the toe of your back foot to the heel of your front foot. Walk this way to the end of the line.**

Scoring: Score pass (+) if the student's feet touch the line with each step, with all steps in a heel-to-toe pattern.

Stationary Balance

Description:
This item assesses the ability to balance the body in a standing position.

Equipment:
- two-inch floor tape
- stopwatch or watch with a second hand

Set Up:
Make a ten-foot tape line on the floor. The student stands on the line facing the examiner.

Directions:
Demonstrate the actions while giving verbal directions. Then repeat the directions without demonstrating. See directions for each skill level.

Trials:
Allow up to three trials for each skill level. If the student demonstrates the actions correctly before the third trial, move on to the next skill level.

Scoring:
Record actual seconds and pass (+) or fail (–) for each level. Score pass (+) if the student demonstrates the task correctly in one of three trials without moving the stationary foot or touching the elevated foot to the floor. Score fail (–) if the student shifts the stationary foot or touches the elevated foot to the floor. Remind the student to keep hands on hips and to keep the raised foot clearly off the floor, but do not record a fail if the student's hands leave the hips or the elevated foot is lowered but does not touch the floor.

RUDIMENTARY: Standing on One Leg for Five Seconds with Eyes Open

Say: **Stand with one foot on the line, place your hands on your hips, lift your other foot off the floor, and look at me. Stand like this until I tell you to stop.**

After five seconds, say *stop*.

*FUNCTIONAL: Standing on One Leg for Ten Seconds with Eyes Open

Say: **Stand with one foot on the line, place your hands on your hips, lift your other foot off the floor, and look at me. Stand like this until I tell you to stop.**

After ten seconds, say *stop*.

MATURE: Standing on One Leg for Ten Seconds with Eyes Closed

Say: **Stand with one foot on the line, place your hands on your hips, lift your other foot off the floor, and close your eyes. Stand like this until I tell you to stop.**

After ten seconds, say *stop*.

Body Roll

Description:
This item assesses the ability to perform a forward roll.

Equipment:
- mat or carpeted surface (optional, but preferred)

Set Up:
The student sits on a mat or floor beside the examiner with knees bent close to chest.

Directions:
Demonstrate the actions while giving verbal directions. Then repeat the directions without demonstrating. See directions for each skill level.

Trials:
Allow up to three trials for each skill level. If the student demonstrates the actions correctly before the third trial, move on to the next skill level.

Scoring:
See directions for each skill level.

RUDIMENTARY: Rocking Forward and Backward

Say: **Sit down, hold knees tight to your chest, tuck your chin against your chest, and rock forward and backward.**

Scoring: Score pass (+) if the student rocks forward and backward at least two times in three trials.

FUNCTIONAL: Beginning Forward Roll Landing in a Sitting Position

Say: **Put your hands on the mat with your arms outside of your knees, tuck your chin against your chest, and place your neck and shoulders on the mat. Roll your body over and land sitting up on the mat.**

Scoring: Score pass (+) if the student rolls completely over and lands in a sitting position at least two times in three trials.

*MATURE: Forward Roll Landing in a Standing Position

Say: **Put your hands on the mat with your arms outside your knees, tuck your chin against your chest, and place your neck and shoulders on the mat. Roll your body forward and land standing up.**

Scoring: Score pass (+) if the student rolls over completely, landing on both feet at least two times in three trials.

Agility

Description:
This item assesses body control while moving, including changing directions, changing speed, starting, stopping, and dodging moving objects.

Equipment:
- two 8- to 10-inch foam or soft rubber balls
- four cones or other stationary objects
- floor tape

Set Up:
Place four cones in a row with five feet between them. Place a two-foot tape line five feet in front of the first cone and another two-foot tape line five feet from the last cone. The student stands on a line facing the cones. After demonstrating, the examiner stands ten feet to the side of the cones to observe the student.

Directions:
Demonstrate the actions while giving verbal directions. Then repeat the directions without demonstrating. See directions for each skill level.

Trials:
Allow up to three trials for each skill level. If the student demonstrates the actions correctly before the third trial, move on to the next skill level.

Scoring:
See directions for each skill level.

RUDIMENTARY: Changing Speed and Direction While Running

Say: **Run slowly in and out of the cones in a figure-eight pattern and then back again without touching the cones. Run fast when I say *fast* and run slow when I say *slow*.**

Give directions to change speed as the student runs.

Scoring: Score pass (+) if the student runs correctly around all cones in a figure-eight pattern without touching them, and responds correctly to instructions for changing speed.

FUNCTIONAL: Starting, Stopping, and Changing Direction While Running

Say: **Run in and out of the cones in a figure-eight pattern and then back again without touching the cones. Stop when I say *stop*, and run again when I say *go*.**

Give directions to start and stop as the student runs.

Scoring: Score pass (+) if the student runs correctly around all cones in a figure-eight pattern without touching them, and stops and starts correctly according to instructions. The student must stop within two steps of hearing the direction to stop.

MATURE: Dodging Moving Objects and Changing Directions While Running

Say: **Run as fast as possible in and out of the cones and then back again without touching the cones. Watch me as you run. I will roll a ball between the cones. Do not touch the rolling ball.**

Roll one ball across the student's path as she or he runs toward the second cone, and roll the other ball as the student runs back.

Scoring: Score pass (+) if the student runs correctly around the cones in a figure-eight pattern without touching the cones or the ball.

Walk

Description:
This item assesses the student's walking pattern.

Equipment:
- none

Set Up:
The student stands 20 feet from the examiner, facing the examiner.

Directions:
Demonstrate the actions while giving verbal directions. Then repeat the directions without demonstrating.

Demonstrate the mature level and then say: **Walk to me**.

Trials:
Administer only three trials for this skill, not three per level.

Scoring:
Score pass (+) for the level of performance (see description for each level below) that best describes the student's walking pattern. Score pass (+) for all levels below that level, and fail (–) for all levels above that level.

RUDIMENTARY: Walking with a Wide Base of Support

Scoring: Score pass (+) if the student holds arms high with bent elbows, leans forward, and takes flat-footed, awkward steps with feet shoulder-width or more apart.

FUNCTIONAL: Walking Flat-Footed

Scoring: Score pass (+) if the student swings arms slightly at waist height in opposition to legs (right arm, left leg-left arm, right leg, etc.), with feet aligned under the shoulders, and takes steps with minimal, slightly awkward heel-to-toe strike.

*MATURE: Walking Smoothly

Scoring: Score pass (+) if the student swings arms at sides in opposition, with feet aligned under the shoulders, and walks with a smoothly integrated heel-to-toe strike.

Horizontal Jump

Description:
This item assesses the ability to perform a horizontal jump, in which the student jumps forward as far as possible, from a bent-knee position.

Equipment:
- mat (optional, but preferred)
- floor tape

Set Up:
Place a one-foot tape line on the floor just in front of the mat. The student stands with toes at the line, facing the mat. The examiner stands to the side of the mat, facing the student.

Directions:
Demonstrate the actions while giving verbal directions. Then repeat the directions without demonstrating.

Demonstrate and then say: **Jump as far as you can.**

Trials:
Administer only three trials for this skill, not three per level.

Scoring:
Score pass (+) for the level of performance (see description for each level below) that best describes the student's horizontal jumping pattern. Score pass (+) for all levels below that level, and fail (–) for all levels above that level.

RUDIMENTARY: Jumping Upward with Uneven Landing

Scoring: Score pass (+) if the student swings arms down and back, jumps more upward than forward with legs moving in front of trunk, and lands awkwardly with one foot before the other.

FUNCTIONAL: Jumping Forward with Arms and Legs Uncoordinated

Scoring: Score pass (+) if the student swings arms and bends knees, jumps more forward than upward with arms and legs moving in a slightly awkward, uncoordinated fashion, and lands on both feet simultaneously.

*MATURE: Jumping Forward with Arms and Legs Coordinated

Scoring: Score pass (+) if the student bends knees, swings arms back and then up above the head, extending body fully by straightening the legs at take off and landing with both feet together, forward of the body.

Vertical Jump

Description:
This item assesses the ability to perform a vertical jump in which the student jumps upward as high as possible from a bent-knee position, extending one arm and touching a wall with the extended arm.

Equipment:

- none

Set Up:
The student stands with her or his side parallel to the wall. The examiner stands facing the wall, about three feet from the student.

Directions:
Demonstrate the actions while giving verbal directions. Then repeat the directions without demonstrating.

Demonstrate as you say: **Stand with your side to the wall. Jump as high as you can. Reach up and touch the wall as high as you can.**

Trials:
Administer only three trials for this skill, not three per level.

Scoring:
Score pass (+) for the level of performance (see description for each level below) that best describes the student's vertical jumping pattern. Score pass (+) for all levels below that level, and fail (−) for all levels above that level.

RUDIMENTARY: Jumping Slightly Upward and Forward with Arms at Sides

Scoring: Score pass (+) if the student stretches his or her body upward incompletely, jumps slightly forward, and moves the arms out at the sides in an awkward, "winging" motion.

FUNCTIONAL: Crouching and Jumping with Arms Above Head

Scoring: Score pass (+) if the student crouches, lifts arms above the head and then to sides, and thrusts the body upward and slightly forward in a slightly awkward fashion.

*MATURE: Jumping with One Arm Extended Upward

Scoring: Score pass (+) if the student stands with feet parallel and shoulder-width apart and the knees bent, reaches one arm upward while the other arm swings sharply downward in opposition, and stretches body fully upward (not forward) during upward jump.

Run

Description:
This item assesses the student's running pattern.

Equipment:
- floor tape

Set Up:
Make two 2-foot tape lines on the floor 20 feet apart.

The student stands with his or her feet behind one of the lines, facing the opposite line. The examiner stands to the side of the lines, near the midpoint, to observe the student's running stride.

Directions:
Demonstrate the actions while giving verbal directions. Then repeat the directions without demonstrating.

Demonstrate a mature run and then say: **Run to the other line.**

Trials:
Administer only three trials for this skill, not three per level.

Scoring:
Score pass (+) for the level of performance (see description for each level below) that best describes the student's running pattern. Score pass (+) for all levels below that level, and fail (–) for all levels above that level.

RUDIMENTARY: Running Flat-Footed with Wide Base of Support

Scoring: Score pass (+) if the student holds arms bent at or above waist height, with feet shoulder-width or wider apart, and takes awkward, short, flat-footed strides with legs slightly bent.

FUNCTIONAL: Running with Arm Opposition and Short Strides

Scoring: Score pass (+) if the student swings arms in opposition below waist but runs with a shorter than normal heel-to-toe stride, with legs bent awkwardly at about a 90-degree angle.

*MATURE: Running with Arm Opposition and Long Strides

Scoring: Score pass (+) if the student swings arms in opposition, and runs with long strides, placing feet in a heel-to-toe pattern, bending the lead leg at about a 90-degree angle.

Hop

Description:
This item assesses the ability to hop forward on one foot while holding the other foot suspended. The student propels himself or herself by bending the knee of the supporting leg and pushing hard and fast upward and forward and landing on the same leg.

Equipment:
- floor tape

Set Up:
Make two 2-foot tape lines on the floor 20 feet apart.

The student stands on one line facing the opposite line. The examiner stands to the side of the lines, near the midpoint, to observe the student's hopping pattern.

Directions:
Demonstrate the actions while giving verbal directions. Then repeat the directions without demonstrating.

Demonstrate a mature hop and then say: **Hop to the other line.**

Trials:
Administer only three trials for this skill, not three per level.

Scoring:
Score pass (+) for the level of performance (see description for each level below) that best describes the quality of the student's hopping pattern. Score pass (+) for all levels below that level, and fail (–) for all levels above that level.

RUDIMENTARY: Hopping with Slight Knee Bend, Minimal Balance

Scoring: Score pass (+) if the student's suspended knee is bent at less than a 90-degree angle, balance is poor, and the arms move excessively and awkwardly.

FUNCTIONAL: Hopping with Full Knee Bend, Exaggerated Arm Swing

Scoring: Score pass (+) if the student's suspended knee is bent at a 90-degree angle, balance is maintained, but the arms swing upward in a slightly awkward manner while hopping.

*MATURE: Hopping with Full Knee Bend, Coordinated Arm Movements

Scoring: Score pass (+) if student's knee is bent at a 90-degree angle, elbows are bent at the sides, and the arms swing slightly at the sides.

Gallop

Description:
This item measures the ability to gallop in which the student leads with one leg and the other leg trails. The lead leg strides forward and the student places his or her weight on that leg while the foot of the trailing leg steps to the heel of the lead leg. Weight is shifted to the trailing leg so that the lead leg can repeat the sequence.

Equipment:
- floor tape

Set Up:
Make two 2-foot tape lines on the floor 20 feet apart.

The student stands behind one line facing the opposite line. The examiner stands to the side of the lines, near the midpoint, to observe the student's galloping pattern.

Directions:
Demonstrate the actions while giving verbal directions. Then repeat the directions without demonstrating.

Demonstrate a mature gallop and then say: **Gallop to the other line.**

Trials:
Administer only three trials for this skill, not three per level.

Scoring:
Score pass (+) for the level of performance (see description for each level below) that best describes the student's galloping pattern. Score pass (+) for all levels below that level, and fail (–) for all levels above that level.

RUDIMENTARY: Galloping Flat-Footed

Scoring: Score pass (+) if the student holds arms bent above the waist, has feet shoulder-width or farther apart, and takes flat-footed, awkward steps leading with one foot and following with the other in short, jerky steps.

FUNCTIONAL: Galloping with Rocking Motion

Scoring: Score pass (+) if the student gallops with knees slightly bent, swings arms at waist level, and lands on the heels in a slightly awkward rocking motion.

*MATURE: Galloping with Long Strides

Scoring: Score pass (+) if the student gallops in long, smooth strides with knees bent and swings arms slightly below the waist in opposition to legs.

Skip

Description:
This item assesses the ability to skip with a rhythmic step-hop pattern.

Equipment:
- floor tape

Set Up:
Make two 2-foot tape lines on the floor 20 feet apart.

The student stands behind one of the lines, facing the opposite line. The examiner stands to the side of the lines, near the midpoint, to observe the student's skipping pattern.

Directions:
Demonstrate the actions while giving verbal directions. Then repeat the directions without demonstrating.

Demonstrate a mature skip and then say: **Skip to the other line.**

Trials:
Administer only three trials for this skill, not three per level.

Scoring:
Score pass (+) for the level of performance (see description for each level below) that best describes the student's skipping pattern. Score pass (+) for all levels below that level, and fail (−) for all levels above that level.

RUDIMENTARY: Skipping Stiffly in a Step-Hop Pattern

Scoring: Score pass (+) if the student skips with an exaggerated step-hop pattern, holding arms stiffly or stationary.

FUNCTIONAL: Skipping with an Exaggerated Airborne Hop

Scoring: Score pass (+) if the student swings arms hard forward and upward, and step-hops in a rhythmical pattern with an exaggerated, slightly awkward, airborne hopping pattern.

*MATURE: Skipping Rhythmically

Scoring: Score pass (+) if the student swings arms slightly in opposition, and step-hops in a relaxed manner with a rhythmic weight transfer from one side to the other.

Arm-Shoulder Flexibility

Description:
This item assesses a student's range of motion or flexibility of the shoulder joint.

Equipment:
- none

Set Up:
The student stands with feet shoulder-width apart, facing the examiner.

Directions:
Demonstrate the actions while giving verbal directions. Then repeat the directions without demonstrating.

Demonstrate mature arm-shoulder flexibility as you say: **Make ten big arm circles.**

Trials:
Administer only three trials for this skill, not three per level.

Scoring:
Score pass (+) for the level of performance (see description for each level below) that best describes the student's arm circles. Score pass (+) for all levels below that level, and fail (–) for all levels above that level.

RUDIMENTARY: Small Arm Circles

Scoring: Score pass (+) if the student holds arms straight out to the side at shoulder level and moves arms in small circles between shoulders and waist.

FUNCTIONAL: Medium Arm Circles

Scoring: Score pass (+) if the student holds arms straight out to the sides at shoulder level and moves arms in medium-sized circles between head and slightly below hips.

*MATURE: Large Arm Circles

Scoring: Score pass (+) if the student holds arms straight out to the side at shoulder level and moves arms in large circles from above head to below hips.

Midbody Flexibility

Description:
This item assesses the range of motion or flexibility of a student's trunk (waist, spine).

Equipment:
- none

Set Up:
The student stands with legs shoulder-width apart and hands on waist, facing the examiner.

Directions:
Demonstrate the mature pattern as you say:

Bend forward as far as possible.
Bend to the side as far as possible.
Bend to the other side as far as possible.
Bend back as far as possible.

Then repeat the directions without demonstrating.

Trials:
Administer only three trials for this skill, not three per level.

Scoring:
Score a pass (+) for the level of performance (see description for each level below) that best describes the student's midbody flexibility. Score pass (+) for all levels below that level, and fail (–) for all levels above that level.

RUDIMENTARY: Slight Trunk Bend

Scoring: Score pass (+) if the student bends slightly in all four directions.

FUNCTIONAL: Moderate Trunk Bend

Scoring: Score pass (+) if the student bends moderately—20 to less than 45 degrees—in all four directions.

*MATURE: Full Trunk Bend

Scoring: Score pass (+) if the student bends fully—45 degrees—in all four directions.

Aerobic Development

Description:
This item assesses a student's heart/lung (aerobic) capacity.

Equipment:
- stopwatch or other timing device

Set Up:
The student jogs in a large area, such as a gym or outdoor practice field.

Directions:
Demonstrate the actions while giving verbal directions. Then repeat the directions without demonstrating.

Demonstrate jogging at an average speed (somewhere between walking and running at full speed) as you say: **Jog as long as you can without stopping.**

Trials:
one

Scoring:
Record the number of minutes of continuous jogging, up to 12 minutes, and score pass (+) for the corresponding level. Score pass (+) for all levels below that level, and fail (–) for all levels above that level.

RUDIMENTARY: One to Four Minutes of Continuous Aerobics at Average Speed

Scoring: Score pass (+) if the student maintains continuous activity for one to four minutes.

FUNCTIONAL: Five to Eight Minutes of Continuous Aerobics at Average Speed

Scoring: Score pass (+) if the student maintains continuous activity for five to eight minutes.

*MATURE: Nine to 12 Minutes of Continuous Aerobics at Average Speed

Scoring: Score pass (+) if the student maintains continuous activity for nine to 12 minutes.

Abdominal Strength

Description:
This item assesses the student's abdominal strength through sit-ups. The student does as many sit-ups as possible in 20 seconds, with knees bent and arms crossed on chest.

Equipment:
- mat
- stopwatch or watch with second hand

Set Up:
The student lies on the mat on his or her back with knees bent at 45-degree angle to floor, feet flat on floor, and arms crossed on chest. The examiner sits or kneels beside the subject.

Directions:
Demonstrate the actions while giving verbal directions. Then repeat the directions without demonstrating.

Demonstrate a sit-up and then say: **When I say *go*, do as many sit-ups as you can until I say *stop*.**

Say *go*.

If necessary, remind student of correct form during each trial. Say *stop* after 20 seconds.

Trials:
one

Scoring:
Record a pass (+) for the level of performance (see description for each level below) that best describes the student's sit-ups. Score pass (+) for all levels below that level, and fail (–) for all levels above that level.

RUDIMENTARY: Sit-Ups at Less Than a 45-Degree Angle with Arms Stretched and Knees Bent

Scoring: Score pass (+) if student does two or more repetitions of less than 45-degrees in poor form with arms uncrossed and legs straightened, stops completely between repetitions, and continues for less than 20 seconds.

FUNCTIONAL: Sit-Ups at 45-Degree Angle for at Least Half of the Sit-Ups, with Arms Crossed and Knees Bent

Scoring: Score pass (+) if student does half or more of the sit-ups in correct form and does continuous repetitions for 20 seconds.

*MATURE: Sit-ups at 45-Degree Angle with Arms Crossed and Knees Bent

Scoring: Score pass (+) if student does nearly all of the sit-ups correctly and does continuous repetitions for 20 seconds.

Leg-Hip Flexibility

Description:
This item assesses a student's range of motion or flexibility of the hip joint.

Equipment:
- none

Set Up:
The student stands with feet shoulder-width apart, facing the examiner.

Directions:
Demonstrate the actions while giving verbal directions. Then repeat the directions without demonstrating.

Demonstrate the mature level of leg-hip flexibility as you say: **Bend over and reach as far as you can toward the floor, keeping your legs straight.**

Trials:
Administer only three trials for this skill, not three per level.

Scoring:
Score a pass (+) for the level of performance (see description of each level below) that best describes the student's leg-hip flexibility. Score pass (+) for all levels below that level, and fail (–) for all levels above that level.

RUDIMENTARY: Touching Fingertips to Toes

Scoring: Score pass (+) if the student stands with legs shoulder-width apart and knees straight and touches toes with fingertips.

FUNCTIONAL: Touching Knuckles to Floor

Scoring: Score pass (+) if the student stands with legs close together and knees straight and touches floor with knuckles.

*MATURE: Touching Palms to Floor

Scoring: Score pass (+) if the student stands with legs close together and knees straight and touches floor with palms of hands.

Arm-Shoulder Strength

Description:
This item assesses a student's arm-shoulder strength through push-ups. The student does full push-ups by lowering chest to fist height, approximately three inches from floor, and supporting the body with hands and toes, with arms extended and back straight in the upright position for up to 20 seconds.

Equipment:
- mat, if available
- stopwatch or watch with a second hand

Set Up:
The student lies on her or his stomach and places both hands flat on mat (or floor) next to the shoulders. The examiner sits or kneels beside the subject.

Directions:
Demonstrate the actions while giving verbal directions. Then repeat the directions without demonstrating.

Demonstrate a mature push-up and then say: **When I say *go*, do as many push-ups as you can until I say *stop*.**

Say *go*.

If necessary, remind the student of the correct form during each trial. Say *stop* after 20 seconds.

Trials:
one

Scoring:
Record a pass (+) for the level of performance (see description of each level below) that best describes the student's sit-ups. Score pass (+) for all levels below that level, and fail (–) for all levels above that level.

RUDIMENTARY: Push-Ups with Elevated Hips

Scoring: Score pass (+) if the student does all repetitions in poor form, with hips raised too high and back not straight, stops between repetitions, and continues for less than 20 seconds.

FUNCTIONAL: Continuous Push-Ups with Adequate Form

Scoring: Score pass (+) if the student does about half of the repetitions in correct form and continues for 20 seconds.

*MATURE: Continuous Push-Ups with Correct Form

Scoring: Score pass (+) if the student does nearly all of the repetitions in correct form and continues for 20 seconds.

Kick

Description:
This item assesses the student's kicking pattern, using a "toe" kick.

Equipment:
- eight- to ten-inch foam, plastic, or rubber ball
- floor tape
- circular target with a ten-inch diameter

Set Up:
Place the target on the wall so that the lowest point of the circumference touches the floor. Make a one-foot tape line on the floor 20 feet from and parallel to the target. Place the ball on the floor about three feet in front of the line. The student stands behind the starting line, three feet from the ball and about 20 feet from the target.

Directions:
Demonstrate the actions while giving verbal directions. Then repeat the directions without demonstrating.

Demonstrate a mature kick as you say: **Kick the ball at the target**.

Trials:
Administer only three trials for this skill, not three per level.

Scoring:
Score a pass (+) for the level of performance (see description for each level below) that best describes the student's kicking pattern. Score pass (+) for all levels below that level, and fail (–) for all levels above that level.

RUDIMENTARY: Kicking Ball with Leg Movement from the Knee

Scoring: Score pass (+) if the student stands near the ball with knee bent and pushes the ball forward awkwardly with the foot, straightening the leg forward after the kick.

FUNCTIONAL: Kicking Ball with Minimal Follow-Through

Scoring: Score pass (+) if the student stands near the ball and straightens the knee before touching the ball, showing little arm-leg opposition and moving the kicking leg forward slightly awkwardly after kicking the ball.

*MATURE: Walking Forward, Stopping, and Kicking Ball with Follow-Through

Scoring: Score pass (+) if the student takes one or more steps toward ball, places support foot near the ball, with arm-leg opposition, straightens the kicking leg before touching the ball, and continues to move the kicking leg forward after kicking the ball.

Bounce/Dribble

Description:
This item assesses the student's ability to bounce and dribble a ten-inch ball.

Equipment:
- ten-inch rubber ball
- two cones
- floor tape

Set Up:
Place two cones in a row, five feet apart. Place a two-foot tape starting line in front of the first cone, about five feet from the cone.

The student stands behind the line, facing the cones. The examiner stands next to the student, behind the starting line.

Directions:
Demonstrate the actions while giving verbal directions. Then repeat the directions without demonstrating. See directions for each skill level.

Trials:
Allow up to three trials for each skill level. If the student demonstrates the actions correctly before the third trial, move on to the next skill level. See directions for each skill level.

Scoring:
See directions for each skill level.

RUDIMENTARY: Bouncing and Trapping Ball with Both Hands

Demonstrate and then say: **Bounce the ball once and catch it.**

> *Scoring*: Score pass (+) if the student stands with feet stationary, shoulder-width apart, holding the ball at about waist height with both hands, and then pushes the ball straight down and traps or catches the bounced ball against the body.

FUNCTIONAL: Dribbling Ball with One Hand, Feet Stationary

Demonstrate and then say: **Stand on the line and use one hand to bounce the ball until I say *stop*.**

Say *stop* after the student bounces the ball continuously for five bounces.

> *Scoring*: Score pass (+) if the student uses one hand to push the ball downward with fingertips, receives bounced ball using the arm, fingers, and wrist, and then continuously pushes the ball back down with one hand for five bounces.

*MATURE: Dribbling Ball with One Hand While Walking or Running

Demonstrate and then say: **Walk or run forward around the cones while you bounce (dribble) the ball with one hand. Then dribble the ball back around the cones to the line.**

> *Scoring*: Score pass (+) if the student pushes the ball downward and forward with fingertips, steps forward as the ball is bounced and uses fingers to continue bouncing it while walking or running forward around the cone and back again, maintaining continuous bouncing while changing directions.

Catch

Description:
This item assesses the student's pattern of catching an eight- to ten-inch ball.

Equipment:
- eight- to ten-inch ball

Set Up:
The student stands facing the examiner, about ten feet away.

Directions:
Demonstrate the actions while giving verbal directions. Then repeat the directions without demonstrating.

Demonstrate a mature catch. (Student can throw the ball to the examiner.) Then say **Catch the ball** as you throw the ball to the student. Toss the ball gently with both hands in an underhand motion directly toward the student so that it arcs from above your waist to above the student's head and then downward toward the student's chest or waist. For the mature level, throw the ball underhand to the student's side so that the student must move about one or two steps to catch it. The ball should be thrown in an arc from waist height to slightly over student's head, so that it reaches the student at about waist height.

Trials:
Allow up to three trials for each skill level. If the student demonstrates the actions correctly before the third trial, move on to the next skill level. See directions for each skill level.

Scoring:
See directions for each skill level.

RUDIMENTARY: Trapping Ball Against Chest with Both Hands

Scoring: Score pass (+) if the student extends arms forward and awkwardly tries to catch the ball with the hands as it approaches by wrapping arms around it and trapping it against the chest.

*FUNCTIONAL: Catching Ball in Both Hands with Feet Stationary

Scoring: Score pass (+) if the student extends bent arms forward, with feet stationary, and catches the ball with hands away from the body.

MATURE: Catching Ball in Both Hands While Moving

Scoring: Score pass (+) if the student extends bent arms forward and moves toward the ball as it is caught, with hands away from the body, and brings ball close to body.

Overhand Throw

Description:
This item assesses the student's ability to throw a ball in an overhand pattern.

Equipment:
- four-inch plastic, foam, yarn, or rubber ball
- floor tape
- circular target (ten-inch diameter)

Set Up:
Place the target on the wall so that the lowest point of the circumference is at the student's eye level. Make a tape line on the floor 20 feet from the target. The student stands behind the line, facing the target. (Student may assume side orientation to target.) The examiner stands beside the student, behind the line.

Directions:
Demonstrate the actions while giving verbal directions. Then repeat the directions without demonstrating.

Demonstrate a mature overhand throw as you say: **Throw the ball overhand at the target.**

Trials:
Administer only three trials for this skill, not three per level.

Scoring:
Score a pass (+) for the level of performance (see description for each level below) that describes the student's overhand throwing pattern. Score pass (+) for all levels below that level, and fail (–) for all levels above that level.

RUDIMENTARY: Throwing Ball Overhand with Feet Stationary

Scoring: Score pass (+) if the student faces the target, keeps feet parallel and stationary, and throws with hand passing over the shoulder or crossing in front of the body diagonally.

FUNCTIONAL: Throwing Ball Overhand While Stepping Forward on the Same Side

Scoring: Score pass (+) if the student faces the target and steps forward with the foot on the same side as the throwing arm, throws the ball with hand passing over shoulder, and follows through with throwing arm.

*MATURE: Throwing Ball Overhand While Stepping Forward on Opposite Side

Scoring: Score pass (+) if the student stands sideways to the target, steps forward with foot opposite throwing arm, and throws ball with hand passing above shoulder and following through with the throwing arm.

Strike

Description:
This item assesses the student's ability to bat a ball with a sidearm motion.

Equipment:
- four- to five-inch (softball size) plastic, foam, or yarn ball
- two plastic bats

Set Up:
The student stands sideways to the examiner, about ten feet away, with feet shoulder-width apart, and holds the bat in both hands over the shoulder that is away from the examiner. The examiner pitches the ball underhand so that it reaches the student at about waist level.

Directions:
Use one of the bats to demonstrate a mature batting pattern. Then say: **Bat the ball when I throw it to you.** Pitch the ball to the student.

Trials:
Allow only three trials for this skill, not three per level. Give extra trials if the ball is not pitched at waist level.

Scoring:
Score a pass (+) for the level of performance (see description for each level below) that describes the student's batting pattern. Score pass (+) for all levels below that level, and fail (–) for all levels above that level.

RUDIMENTARY: Swinging Bat with Feet Stationary

Scoring: Score pass (+) if the student grips the bat with hands together about one inch from the base, one hand on top of the other, holds bat out to the side with elbows slightly bent, stands almost sideways to the ball, and swings the bat down and across the front of the body awkwardly, keeping feet stationary without transferring body weight.

FUNCTIONAL: Swinging Bat and Transferring Weight

Scoring: Score pass (+) if the student grips the bat with hands together about one inch from the base, one hand on top of the other, holds the bat up and back over shoulder, stands sideways to the ball, and swings the bat down and horizontally while transferring weight to the lead foot.

*MATURE: Swinging Bat, Transferring Weight, and Following Through

Scoring: Score pass (+) if the student grips the bat with hands together about one inch from the base, dominant hand on top, holds the bat over the shoulder, stands sideways to the ball with weight on the foot farthest from ball, swings the bat forward leading with the hands and shifts weight to the forward foot in a smooth, integrated motion.

Underhand Throw

Description:
This item assesses the student's underhand throwing pattern.

Equipment:
- four-inch plastic, foam, or yarn ball
- floor tape
- circular wall target (ten-inch diameter)

Set Up:
Place the target on the wall so that the lowest point of circumference is at the student's eye level. Make a one-foot tape line 20 feet from and parallel to the target. The student stands behind the line facing the target.

Directions:
Demonstrate the actions while giving verbal directions. Then repeat the directions without demonstrating.

Demonstrate a mature underhand throw as you say: **Throw the ball underhand at the target.**

Trials:
Administer only three trials for this skill, not three per level.

Scoring:
Score pass (+) for the level of performance (see description for each level below) that describes the student's underhand throwing pattern. Score pass (+) for all levels below that level, and fail (−) for all levels above that level.

RUDIMENTARY: Throwing Ball Underhand with Feet Stationary

Scoring: Score pass (+) if the student stands with feet shoulder-width apart, swings the throwing arm downward, back, and then forward, and releases the ball without following through with the throwing arm.

FUNCTIONAL: Throwing Ball Underhand While Stepping Forward on the Same Side

Scoring: Score pass (+) if the student swings the throwing arm downward, back, and then forward, while stepping forward on the same side, releases ball and follows through with the throwing arm.

*MATURE: Throwing Ball Underhand While Stepping Forward with Opposite Foot

Scoring: Score pass (+) if the student swings the throwing arm forward and up, and then swings the throwing arm downward, back, and then forward while stepping forward with the opposite foot, releases the ball, and follows through with the throwing arm.

Underhand Roll

Description:
This item assesses the student's ability to roll a ball using an underhand motion.

Equipment:
- seven-inch foam, rubber, or plastic ball

Set Up:
The student stands facing the examiner, 20 feet away. The examiner stands facing the student.

Directions:
Demonstrate the actions while giving verbal directions. Then repeat the directions without demonstrating.

Demonstrate a mature underhand roll and then say: **Roll the ball to me.**

Trials:
Administer only three trials for this skill, not three per level.

Scoring:
Score a pass (+) for the level of performance (see description for each skill level below) that describes the student's underhand rolling pattern. Score pass (+) for all levels below that level, and fail (−) for all levels above that level.

RUDIMENTARY: Rolling Ball from Between Legs in Standing Position

Scoring: Score pass (+) if the student stands leaning forward with feet shoulder-width apart and knees bent, holds the ball with hands on the side and the back of the ball, and then swings the ball slightly back and pushes it forward, extending both arms.

FUNCTIONAL: Rolling Ball from Side in Standing Position

Scoring: Score pass (+) if the student stands with feet apart and holds the ball in both hands at about waist height, and then swings the ball down and back to one side, mainly with one hand, while bending knees and leaning forward, releases the ball with one hand, and follows through with hand and arm, shifting weight to one side, but not from one leg to another.

*MATURE: Rolling Ball from Side While Stepping with Opposite Leg and Transferring Weight

Scoring: Score pass (+) if the student stands with feet close together holding ball in both hands at about waist height, swings the ball down and back on one side with one hand while bending the knees and leaning forward, steps forward with the foot opposite the rolling arm, releases the ball, and follows through with the rolling arm.

Small-Object Control

Description:
This item assesses the student's skill in manipulating small objects through stacking blocks. The student is asked to stack six blocks to make a vertical tower.

Equipment:
- six small blocks
- table

Set Up:
Place six blocks on the table. The student sits at the table facing the examiner.

Directions:
Demonstrate how to stack blocks to build a tower and then say: **Stack the blocks directly on top of one another to make a tower.**

Trials:
one

Scoring:
Score a pass (+) for the level of performance (see description for each level below) that describes the student's performance. Score pass (+) for all levels below that level, and fail (–) for all levels above that level.

RUDIMENTARY: Stacking Two Blocks in Uneven Alignment

Scoring: Score pass (+) if the student stacks two blocks, but the blocks are not placed directly on top of one another.

FUNCTIONAL: Stacking Three Blocks in Straight Alignment

Scoring: Score pass (+) if the student stacks at least three blocks in a tower, fairly well aligned and firmly positioned.

*MATURE: Stacking Six Blocks in Straight Alignment

Scoring: Score pass (+) if the student stacks six blocks in a neat, well-balanced tower.

Grasp

Description:
This item assesses the student's ability to grasp objects.

Equipment:

- a small object that is easy to grasp with the palm of one hand and has some motivational qualities, such as a brightly colored toy, ball, or block
- table

Set Up:
The student sits at a table; the object is placed on the table in front of the student.

Directions:
Demonstrate a mature grasp, showing the student how to pick up the object. Then say: **Pick up the toy (ball).**

Trials:
Administer only three trials for this skill, not three per level.

Scoring:
Score a pass (+) for the level of performance (see description of each level below) that describes the student's grasp. Score pass (+) for all levels below that level, and fail (−) for all levels above that level.

RUDIMENTARY: Reaching for and Touching Object

Scoring: Score pass (+) if the student reaches for the object with one hand and touches it.

FUNCTIONAL: Grasping Object in Palm

Scoring: Score pass (+) if the student reaches for the object, grasps it with the entire hand, and picks it up.

*MATURE: Grasping Object with Thumb and Forefinger

Scoring: Score pass (+) if the student reaches for the object, grasps it with the thumb and forefinger in a pincer hold, and picks it up.

Hand Strength

Description:
This item assesses a student's hand strength while squeezing a soft object.

Equipment:
- two-inch yarn, foam, or newspaper ball
- stopwatch or watch with second hand

Set Up:
The student sits facing the examiner.

Directions:
Show the student how to squeeze the ball as hard as possible in the palm of your hand. Then say: **Squeeze the ball as long as you can or until I say stop.**

After 30 seconds, say *stop*.

Trials:
one

Scoring:
Score a pass (+) for the level of performance (see description of each level below) that describes the student's hand strength. Score pass (+) for all levels below that level, and fail (–) for all levels above that level.

RUDIMENTARY: Squeezing Ball for Ten Seconds

Scoring: Score pass (+) if the student squeezes the ball continuously for ten seconds.

FUNCTIONAL: Squeezing Ball for 20 Seconds

Scoring: Score pass (+) if the student squeezes the ball continuously for 20 seconds.

*MATURE: Squeezing Ball for 30 Seconds

Scoring: Score pass (+) if the student squeezes the ball continuously for 30 seconds.

Visual-Motor Control

Description:
This item assesses the student's ability to copy a cross and a five-pointed star.

Equipment:
- page 7 of MSI Record Booklet
- pencil
- table

Set Up:
The student sits at a table holding a pencil with page 7 of the MSI Record Book.

Directions:
Say: **Look at the shape in this box. Make one just like it in the empty box below.**

Trials:
one

Scoring:
Precision of shape is the primary criterion used for scoring. Guidelines for judging precision are outlined for each level below. Details and examples are included with the specific criteria for each drawing.

Rudimentary. The drawing does not resemble the standard, contains extraneous lines, or has missing parts.

Consider as extraneous those lines that have no relationship to the shape of the drawing. Do not consider as extraneous lines that result from an overlap or lines that extend slightly.

Examples:

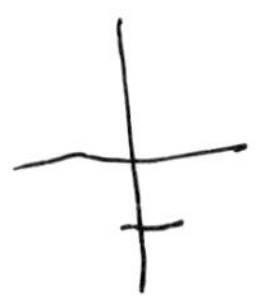

extraneous line

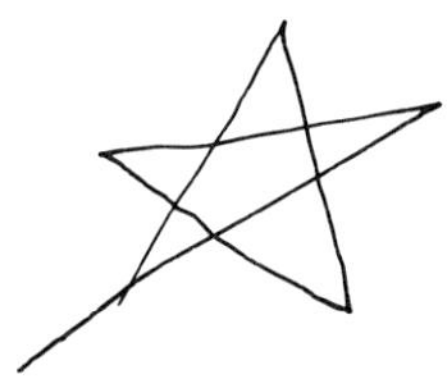

extended line

Functional. The drawing resembles the general shape of the standard, includes all lines, and contains no extraneous lines, though some lines may be slightly short, overlapping, or extended.

Mature. The drawing closely resembles the standard in exactness of its lines, general proportion, and configuration. It includes all lines and contains no extraneous lines.

Copying a Cross

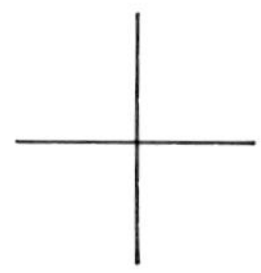

Standard

RUDIMENTARY

Scoring: Score a plus (+) if

—the drawing is comprised of more or fewer than two lines.

—the drawing has two lines which fail to cross each other completely.

—the drawing is larger than the space provided or less than 1/2 the size of standard.

Examples:

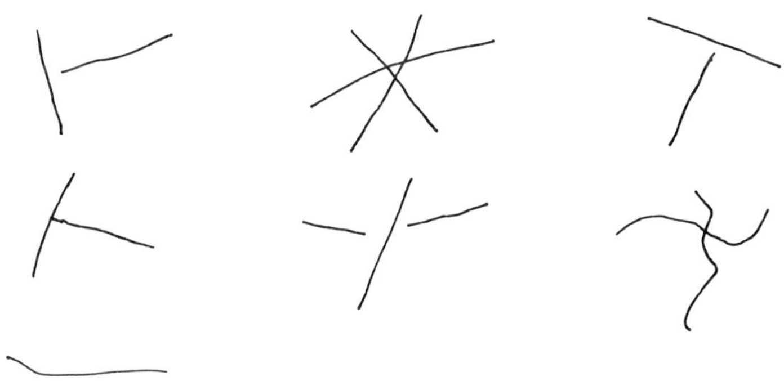

FUNCTIONAL

Scoring: Score a plus (+) if

—the drawing is comprised of two relatively straight lines that completely cross each other at some point.

—the drawing is not larger than the space provided or less than 1/4 the size of standard.

Examples:

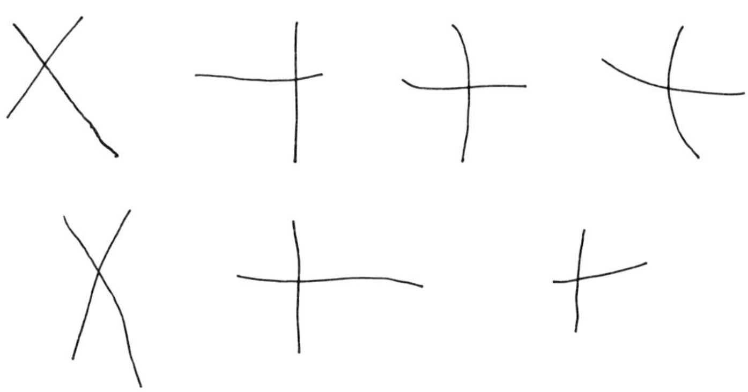

MATURE

Scoring: Score a plus (+) if

—the drawing has two straight lines of approximately the same length (one line is not more that 1 1/2 times the length of the other line).

—the drawing has straight lines which cross each other completely at approximately right angles (between 75 degrees and 105 degrees).

—the drawing has straight lines which cross each other approximately at their midpoints (within 1/4 inch of the midpoints of each).

Examples:

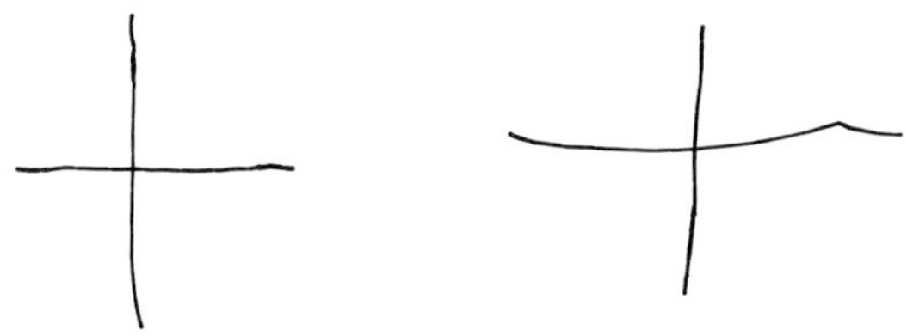

Copying a Star

Standard

RUDIMENTARY

Scoring: Score plus (+) if

—the drawing has fewer or more than five lines.

—the drawing does not have five definite outside points.

—the drawing does not have five definite inside corners.

—the drawing is larger than space provided or less than 1/2 the size of the standard.

—the drawing has extended lines of more than 1/4 inch at the points of the star.

Examples:

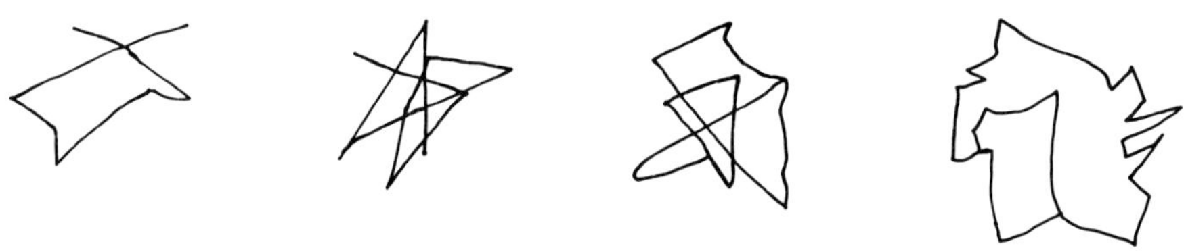

FUNCTIONAL

Scoring: Score plus (+) if

—the drawing resembles a five-pointed star composed of five relatively straight lines.

—the drawing has five definite outside points and five definite inside corners (lines must meet at points).

—the drawing is not larger than space provided or less than 1/2 the size of the standard.

—the drawing has no more than one extended line of more than 1/4 inch at the points.

Examples:

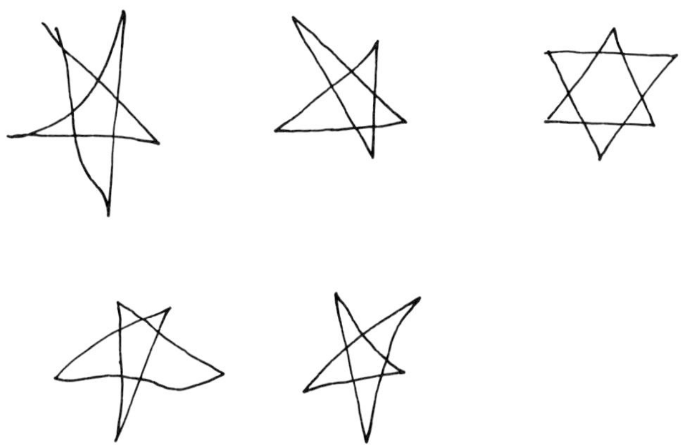

MATURE

Scoring: Score plus (+) if

—the drawing closely resembles the standard with angles forming five points of moderate size (none is less than 15 degrees or more than 75 degrees).

—the angles forming the five points are of approximately the same size.

—the five points are all approximately the same length, (none is more than 1 1/4 times the length of any other).

—the drawing has no gaps and/or overlapping lines of more than 1/8 inch.

Examples:

Appendix B

Adaptations for Students with Handicapping Conditions

The *Body Skills* curriculum is designed for teachers to use when instructing preschool through elementary-age students with a wide range of ability in performing motor skills. The developmental sequences presented on the skill folders and in the Motor Skills Inventory (MSI) are based on the sequence of motor skill development in average children, but the activities are designed to be flexible to meet the needs of all children, including those with handicapping conditions.

The *Body Skills* curriculum can be modified to accommodate the needs of students with handicaps. A number of adaptations that may be made in instructional procedures or the environment are listed on the backs of the skill folders. This appendix presents an overview of particular handicapping conditions and additional adaptations that may be made for students with these conditions.

Instruction should be planned with careful consideration for the characteristics and unique needs of each student. The assessment process using the *Bruininks-Oseretsky Test* and the MSI helps in gathering information about the skill levels of students in the class. The assessment results, however, often do not provide enough information to develop a plan to meet the needs of all students. Skill-based assessment alone is not adequate for determining all the important, unique characteristics and handicaps of students. Information about handicapping conditions must be gathered from informal assessment procedures, examination of student records (for example, health and diagnostic information), and discussions with the student's family and appropriate professionals. Not all conditions have an effect on performance in physical activities. A formal assessment in addition to informal assessment information may help reveal a more complete picture of the potential impact a student's disability may have on performance in various motor activities.

Instructing students with handicaps in physical activities requires special planning and preparation. Many disabilities impose limitations on the extent to which students can participate in physical activities. In planning to use the *Body Skills* curriculum with students with handicaps, it is important to review the health status of each student with school nurses and to consult, as needed, with parents or guardians to ensure that students can participate in the activities without personal injury. It may be important, for example, to confer with special education teachers, physical therapists, occupational therapists, health personnel, and others regarding a student's limitations and any adaptations that may be needed for physical activities.

Teachers working with students who are taking medication for handicapping conditions need to check each student's medication and medication schedule and to understand possible side effects of the medication. The activities may need to be modified around the medication or its side effects.

The philosophy of the *Body Skills* program is that students with handicaps should participate in physical activities with nonhandicapped peers. The activities can, of course, be used for specialized adaptive physical education programs, but the content and format of activities provide rich opportunities for social integration of handicapped students. One possible strategy is to encourage all students to work together in redesigning the activity to facilitate greater social integration of students with handicaps.

Participation in the *Body Skills* activities provides unique opportunities for students with handicaps to improve self-concepts and to develop positive attitudes about participating in physical activities. To this end, teachers must emphasize that students are competing only with themselves. This may be done through the use of the Individual Skill Progress Checklist and through informally charting individual progress through the individual practice activities. In an atmosphere of acceptance and encouragement, students with handicaps may discover recreational activities that can be enjoyed throughout life.

The following adaptations are grouped according to type of handicapping condition: emotional and behavior disorders, hearing impairments, learning disabilities, mental retardation, physical impairments, and visual impairment. The adaptations for each handicapping condition are organized into instructional and environmental categories. Instructional adaptations include variations in the length of an activity, altering directions when teaching an activity, and/or specific suggestions for modifying the strategies in the activity. Environmental adaptations refer to modifications that can be made in the teaching setting or the equipment.

Emotional and Behavior Disorders

Emotional disturbance is a generic term describing a variety of personality characteristics and disorders. Public Law 94-142 describes serious emotional disturbance as a condition existing over a long period of time that to a marked degree adversely affects educational performance and exhibits one or more of the following characteristics:

An inability to learn which cannot be explained by intellectual, sensory, or health factors.

An inability to build or maintain satisfactory interpersonal relationships with peers and teachers.

Inappropriate types of behavior or feelings under normal circumstances.

A general pervasive mood of unhappiness or depression.

A tendency to develop physical symptoms or fears associated with personal or school problems (Public Law 94-142 1975).

Implications for physical activity among students with emotional or behavior disorders differ according to their specific problems. The teacher must have a thorough understanding and working knowledge of the student's characteristics, appropriate background information, and current educational plan.

Instructional Adaptations

- Reward and praise demonstrations of appropriate behavior.
- Use behavior modification techniques to reinforce acceptable and cooperative behavior; techniques used should be consistent among all teachers and parents.
- Avoid conflict and power struggles by separating students who do not get along well with each other; always reinforce strategies of cooperation.

- Explain the purpose of physical contact in activities to avoid misinterpretation by students.
- Give consideration to the student's social skills when selecting activities—the student may have the skills to work with one peer, but not a team of six peers.
- Demonstrate appropriate ways of showing anger.
- Teach the student how to read social cues and body language.
- Appoint the student to be leader. Use the student's name frequently.
- Establish and enforce a few clear, strict rules with appropriate meaningful consequences for the student; for example, "If you step over the line before I say go, then you must go to the end of the line."

Environmental Adaptations

- Carefully structure the environment to eliminate distractions for easily excited and distractible students.

Hearing Impairments

Auditory handicaps are one of the most common disabilities affecting children. They range from slight deviation from normal hearing to total loss of sound perception. The term *hearing-impaired* describes all hearing disorders that deviate from normal, including deafness.

The most obvious adjustment for a child with a hearing impairment is the loss of a normal mode of communication. If the loss of hearing is congenital or acquired before speech has been learned, a means of conveying as well as receiving information must be learned.

The majority of hearing-impaired students possess average motor abilities. Motor deficiencies or developmental delay usually result from minimal opportunity to play with other children. It is essential that hearing-impaired students be provided with the opportunity to experience stimulating movement experiences and physical activity.

Instructional Adaptations

- Be sure the student can see demonstrations. Use other students or an interpreter to give instructions in sign language.
- Draw attention to details in movement patterns by pointing out joints (for example, marking joints with ribbons) and using visual illustrations and other cues.
- Have a highly skilled student demonstrate actions while you point out specific details of the movements.
- Preteach signs and signals specific to particular actions before the activity.
- Face the student while teaching, using eye contact, gestures, and facial expression.

Environmental Adaptations

- Use mirrors to draw attention to the student's performance and form.
- Use color-coded or brightly colored equipment.

- Provide strong picture cues for the student. Encourage the student to pay attention to the vibrations created by sounds in music, locomotor skills, and ball bouncing; for example, allow the student to touch an audio player to feel the vibrations.
- Use flags, flashing lights, signs, and posters to communicate directions to the student.

Learning Disabilities

According to Public Law 94-142, a learning disability is a disorder in one or more of the basic psychological processes involved in understanding or in using spoken or written language. The disorder may manifest itself in the difficulty to listen, think, speak, read, write, spell, or do mathematics. A learning-disabled student possesses normal potential and opportunity, yet a significant discrepancy exists between the student's achievement and academic ability (Public Law 94-142 1975). Students with learning disabilities possess normal or above average intelligence; thus, a learning-disabled student can fulfill his or her learning potential provided that the student's unique learning needs are understood and accommodated.

Five learning/behavioral disorders that have implications for physical activity:

Distractibility: Inability to focus attention on appropriate tasks. A typical learning environment is often overstimulating.

Disinhibition: Random shifts in attention and daydreaming.

Hyperactivity: Displaying excess energy or seeming always in motion.

Perseveration: Inability to stop an activity once it has begun.

Social Imperception: Inappropriate social behavior and inability to comprehend the meaning of one's own actions or the actions of others.

To meet the needs of students with learning disabilities and attention problems during physical activities, it is imperative to understand the unique learning characteristics of the student. The physical activity settings should be structured to guarantee success for the student in the initial stages of learning activities. Physical activity can provide a unique opportunity for the learning disabled student to feel positive about his or her abilities and to develop social skills necessary to function successfully in regular education environments.

Adaptations

For Hyperactive Students:

- Provide highly structured activities and directions with consistent routines from day to day.
- Use color or sound, or eliminate irrelevant stimuli and unnecessary equipment, to keep the student's attention.
- Use mirrors to highlight and focus on the student's movements.
- Organize and structure physical space. Have the student move in a small space. Use lane or space markers to define space.

For Students Who Perseverate:

- Plan a sequence of activities in which each part is distinctly different from the others.

- Have the student sit down or go to a specific spot or position between parts of the activity.
- Use stop-and-go activities.

For Students Who Lack Social Perceptiveness:

- Teach the student to read social cues, voice intonations, and body language.
- Impose considerable structure on the activity.
- Pair the student with students who have good social and interpersonal skills.
- Emphasize strategies to enhance memory of steps and actions in activities through frequent short practice sessions, testing of concepts, and repeating rules and concepts in sentences.

Other Adaptations:

- Use various group formations to emphasize the student's role as part of the entire group.
- Give frequent reminders of the sequence in the activity to aid in establishing a routine.
- Use cones or flags to delineate boundaries for activities.
- Obtrusively mark right and left limbs for students who are confused about right and left.

Mental Retardation

Mental retardation is defined as significantly subaverage general intellectual functioning, existing concurrently with deficits in adaptive behavior, and manifested during the developmental period, which adversely affects a student's educational performance (Grossman 1983). The common characteristic of students whose development is retarded is substantial difficulty in learning. Although physical handicaps are more common among children classified as mentally retarded, most are ambulatory and do not have substantial health conditions.

Generally, mentally retarded students achieve below age-level in motor proficiency, but many students often surpass the performance averages of their normal, chronological age peers (Bruininks 1974). Because mentally retarded persons are more like their normal peers in physical motor ability than in any other respect, the role of physical activity in educational programs is very important.

Physical activity offers students who are retarded an opportunity for social integration with nonhandicapped peers and provides excellent opportunities for learning leisure activities and motor skills related to vocational success and community integration.

Instructional Adaptations

- Use short, clear statements when giving instructions.
- Choose activities that are age and socially appropriate.
- Follow a consistent routine when teaching.
- Break down the skill into smaller increments if initial attempts at learning activities are not successful.
- Provide multiple cues by using clear verbal instructions, clear demonstrations of correct performance, and by providing manual guidance if needed, for the student to practice the skill pattern.

- Provide short, spaced opportunities for practice to give ample opportunities to experience success and to maintain motivation.
- Provide one-to-one preteaching prior to the activity to help in skill acquisition and success during the activity. Repeat performance of the skill and the activity rules through individual practice sessions.
- Pair the student with a more-able peer who will give assistance during the activity.
- Be sure the student is paying attention before giving direction. Use visual illustrations and demonstrations using peers.
- Provide prior teaching of the vocabulary to be used during the activity.
- Emphasize strategies to enhance memory of steps and actions in activities through frequent short practice sessions, testing of concepts, and memory strategies, such as repeating rules and concepts in sentences.

Environmental Adaptations

- Use brightly colored equipment and materials to help focus students' attention.
- Use music and rhythm to establish patterns of movement as often as possible.

Physical Impairments (Ambulatory and Nonambulatory)

Arthritis

Arthritis is inflammation of the joints. It is also a "hidden" handicap because the damage and pain are not readily visible to others. Conditions common to arthritis include atrophy of various muscle groups, postural abnormalities, swollen and painful joints, and other symptoms resulting from medications. A deceptive and misunderstood aspect of arthritis is the fact that it is erratic and unpredictable; it may change from day to day or even from morning to afternoon. A student may have minimal pain or stiffness one day, yet on the next day, may not be able to move without experiencing severe pain.

Physical activity can be very valuable for the student with arthritis. Participation in physical activity helps to lessen and prevent joint stiffness and can provide psychological benefits. Proper judgment as to when to exercise and when to rest is very critical. Because exercise during flare-ups can result in irreversible joint damage, teachers, physicians, and parents should work together to develop guidelines for activity schedules.

Instructional Adaptations

- Avoid long periods of sitting or lying still.
- Conduct frequent short periods of activity approximately three times a day rather than one long exercise period.
- Teach easy skills or activities when the student is experiencing flare-ups. If an activity causes the student pain, substitute activities that use different movements and do not cause pain.
- Use slow, easy warm-up and cool-down stretches before and after activities.
- Require alternative skills or movements if running, jumping, and leaping are difficult for the student to perform.
- Allow frequent rest periods.
- Emphasize extension and smoothness in all muscle movements.

- Avoid jarring and jamming of any body parts.
- Provide a home program and keep the student updated on rules and activities during homebound periods.
- Schedule physical activity in the late morning or afternoon.

Environmental Adaptations

- Teach skills and activities in a swimming pool.
- Use a tricycle when appropriate to keep joints mobile without jarring or jamming.
- See that the gymnasium is reasonably warm to keep the student's joints flexible.
- Use lightweight equipment and mats to soften the surface.

Cardiovascular Disorders

Cardiovascular disorders include all diseases of the heart and blood vessels. Restrictions vary for students with cardiovascular disorders. Many students are able to exercise freely or compete in organized athletics, whereas other students will be forced to limit their participation. Communication with parents and the family physician is important when initially planning the physical activity program. Any restrictions and limits on physical activity should be stated in the student's program. Progress slowly with the student and consult the physician and therapist periodically. If necessary, incorporate the physician's recommendations for post-operative exercises into the activity.

Instructional Adaptations

- Slow the pace of the activity. Encourage the student to stop when fatigued, and never push the student.
- Have the student perform exercises while lying or sitting, where appropriate in the activities.
- Frequently take the student's pulse rate. Know the student's resting heart rate and obtain baseline pulse measures in various situations. Make the activity easier if the heart rate does not return to resting rate within three minutes.
- Always have the student exercise with a partner, taking each other's pulse rate and monitoring the intensity of exercise.
- Rotate the student's positions frequently (for example, from offense to defense, from sitting out to playing a front line, from side line to back line) to moderate the intensity of the activities.
- Limit activity during hot or humid weather.
- Reduce emotional stress and competition by helping the student keep calm and not become too agitated.
- Use mild strength-building activities with lightweight equipment and light low-impact aerobics.
- Modify the rules of the activity to eliminate any rigorous body contact and activity levels that are too strenuous.

Environmental Adaptations

- Provide mats for frequent rest periods.
- Use a metronome beat to encourage pacing.
- Assign a smaller space or limit the distance the student must move.

Cerebral Palsy

Cerebral palsy is characterized by paralysis, weakness, incoordination, and/or other motor dysfunctions caused by damage to the motor area of the brain. Basic classifications of cerebral palsy include:

Monoplegia—involving one limb

Triplegia—involving three limbs (usually the legs and one arm)

Quadriplegia—involving all four extremities

Hemiplegia—involving the arm and leg on one side of the body.

The six types of cerebral palsy are

Spasticity—characterized by muscle movements that are explosive, jerky, poorly coordinated, and sometimes unpredictable.

Athetosis—characterized by slow, involuntary, uncontrollable twisting movements of the extremities. Children with this type of cerebral palsy are constantly moving in unpredictable and purposeless motion, with common associated disorders in hearing, speech, and vision.

Ataxia—a disorder of balance and posture characterized by a lack of gross and fine motor coordination. Movements are slow and deliberate, yet awkward. Walking is difficult, typically characterized by lurching, lunging, and frequent falling.

Rigidity—characterized by hypertensity of both agonist and antagonist muscles, making movement very difficult.

Tremor—characterized by uncontrolled, involuntary rhythmic movements. The tremor is usually increased with voluntary movements. This type of cerebral palsy occurs quite infrequently.

A multidisciplinary approach is advised in planning physical activity programs for students with cerebral palsy. It is important that therapists, physical educators, and teachers coordinate their efforts to enhance the effectiveness of services. Students must be trained in proper techniques of beneficial stretching specific to their individual needs for beginning physical activities. Flexibility activities in the Body Fitness module may be used to promote stretching.

The *Body Skills* program provides a unique opportunity for students with cerebral palsy to improve their body image, posture, flexibility, and locomotion and to develop motor strength and positive attitudes about participating in physical activities.

Instructional Adaptations

- Spend five to ten minutes doing relaxed stretching of arms, legs, trunk, and neck before beginning physical activities. Incorporate frequent stretching into the activities (such as reaching for equipment or bending to pick up objects). Teach the student to stretch on her or his own to increase flexibility for physical activities.
- Allow plenty of time for the student to perform the skill or activity, allowing him or her to repeat the skill or parts of the skill.
- Adjust the skill requirements to the student's joint and muscle strength and flexibility.
- Pair the student with a partner whose skills complement the student's abilities.

Environmental Adaptations

- Use lightweight balls.
- Use velcro straps, special grips, or gloves to assist the student in gripping the equipment.
- Use scooters, walkers, or other assistive devices to aid mobility.
- Ask the student to wear light weights on wrists or ankles to help stretch tight muscles.
- Use brightly colored equipment to mark boundaries, so students will see them when they are moving.
- When teaching new skills, additional support can be provided by having the student lean or hold onto a chair, a rail, or the wall.
- Place a firm hand on the student's shoulder to help steady him or her during physical movements.

Epilepsy

Epilepsy is defined as sudden alterations of brain functions and consciousness that usually result in a brief period of impaired consciousness or seizure. Seizures occur because the brain is overwhelmed with an abundance of nerve activity.

Epilepsy is a common condition that is treated and controlled with medication. The majority of students with epilepsy are able to participate in physical activity without limitations, provided that common sense and basic safety guidelines are followed. It is important that students with epilepsy not be overprotected and be allowed to participate in physical activities to develop self-confidence and a positive self-image.

Instructional Adaptations

- Avoid conditions that have been known to precede seizures for the student. These conditions may include high levels of stress, hyperventilation, contact activities.
- Teach proper breathing techniques during the activity. Avoid or alter activities that require students to hold their breath.
- Teach relaxation techniques.
- Stand next to and observe the student closely for extended periods when he or she is first learning a new motor skill.

Environmental Adaptations

- Use a carpeted surface and equipment made of sponge or foam.
- Use equipment that is close to the ground or floor.
- Have the student wear protective head gear, if needed.
- Avoid conditions that have been known to precede seizures for the student. These conditions may include flashing lights or heights.

Missing Limbs

Absence of limbs may be congenital or acquired. The effect on motor skill development depends on the limb and severity of amputation.

One of the most important considerations for a student with a missing limb is the development of a positive self-image. Students are often very self-conscious of even slight differences in their bodies; an amputation may present particular difficulties with an individual's positive self-image and self-confidence.

Physical activities and exercises should be planned in consultation with the family physician for students with special physical disabilities. Maintaining proper range of motion of all joints, including the affected limb, is vital to development. Muscle strength development will facilitate adequate control of the prosthesis or maximum use of a crutch or cane.

Problems with balance are common among children with missing limbs. The teacher should provide opportunities for students to experience physical activities that help them adjust to the change in the center of gravity in response to the missing limb. Physical activity should be a high priority in the student's educational plan to increase physical activity and to control weight. It is important that the student participate in activities in which she or he will be physically active, experience success, and improve self-image.

Instructional Adaptations

- Preteach skills in the instructional setting using the individual practice suggestions.
- Change the skill requirements to fit the student's capabilities.
- Substitute skills the student needs to practice for skills called for in the activity to enable participation on an adjusted basis.
- Allow the student to play a position in which movement is confined to a small area.
- Allow the student more time, steps, rolls, or support in order to perform the desired skills.
- Adjust the rules for activities. For example, in an activity in which students must reach a goal line, give the student credit if any part of the student's body or assistive device crosses the line.
- Adjust activities to provide more limited roles for students with disabilities. For example, require nonhandicapped students to move in a more difficult manner, such as backward or in a crab walk or crawl.

Environmental Adaptations

- Shorten the distance for the student.
- Use walkers, tricycles, scooters, crutches, parallel bars, bars, or carts with wheels to aid mobility.
- Provide additional support and balance to students during the activity.
- Extend the student's reach with floor hockey sticks, rackets, or paddles.
- Teach skills and activities in a swimming pool to counteract the effects of gravity.

Muscular Dystrophy

Muscular dystrophy is the progressive degeneration of the skeletal or voluntary muscles caused by muscle-cell deterioration. Adaptations of physical activity will depend on the type of muscular dystrophy and how far the disease has progressed. It is important to maintain cardiovascular fitness through participation in activities such as swimming or vigorous inhale/exhale exercises, including blowing up balloons, blowing out candles, blowing Ping-Pong balls across a table, or blowing bubbles. The student with muscular dystrophy should participate with other students whenever possible to increase social interaction and self-confidence. Physical activity provides students with muscular dystrophy enjoyment as well as a chance to develop leisure skills.

Instructional Adaptations

- Increase and/or prolong movement as long as possible in activities requiring locomotion.
- Provide frequent periods of activity, as much as the student can tolerate, with small achievements; for example, moving only a few feet instead of across the entire room. Encourage the student to participate as vigorously as possible, but allow for frequent rests.
- Assign the student a smaller area of movement.
- Assign a student buddy to help with those parts of an activity the student is unable to do without assistance. Pair the student with a buddy who can complement the student's weaknesses and allow the student with the disability to contribute his or her own best skills.

Environmental Adaptations

- Use braces, crutches, other assistive devices, such as scooters or wheelchairs, to aid mobility.
- Teach skills and activities in a swimming pool to counteract the effects of gravity.
- Provide light, easily gripped foam or sponge equipment.
- Use velcro straps, special grips, or gloves to assist the student in gripping the equipment.

Respiratory Diseases

Common respiratory diseases include asthma, allergies, and cystic fibrosis. With proper supervision and planning, students with respiratory diseases can participate successfully in physical activities.

Respiratory diseases vary in levels of severity. For some students, restriction is necessary only when the condition flares up; for other students, full restriction and limited activity are necessary. Students with respiratory diseases may be motorically delayed as a result of limited exposure to physical activity and play restrictions. Acquisition of motor skills should be a priority in the educational plan for students with respiratory diseases, with particular emphasis placed on recreational activities that can be enjoyed throughout life.

Instructional Adaptations

- Build the student's tolerance by using the performance one day as the goal to meet or exceed the next day, concentrating on mild activity for 10 to 15 minutes a day.
- Alternate frequent short rests with frequent periods of short exercise to build tolerance.
- Monitor the student's heart rate and respirations to obtain a baseline rate of involvement in activities, and plan the student's program to build upon that base level.
- Consult music specialists to aid in teaching correct breathing patterns. Emphasize inhale and exhale patterns during exercise.
- Use activities that build the student's upper-body strength.
- Reduce stress in activities by reducing competition.
- Teach relaxation skills to the student instead of vigorous movement.

- Have the student practice blowing up balloons, blowing out candles, or blowing Ping-Pong balls across a floor or across water.
- Include swimming to enhance respiratory capacity.
- Allow the student to walk rather than run during movement activities.

Environmental Adaptations

- Use a metronome to aid the student in pacing herself or himself.
- Use indoor activities if outdoor breathing exhausts the student.
- Provide tissues and wastebaskets in the activity area.

Spinal Cord Injuries

A spinal cord injury is a permanent injury to the spinal cord nerves that stimulate and control the skeletal muscles. When a spinal cord injury occurs, muscle paralysis below the injury site results. Usually, the higher the injury site, the more prevalent the damage and loss of muscle function.

A spinal cord injury may be complete, resulting in total loss of function, or it may be partial, resulting in some functional muscle control. An injury in the cervical vertebrae (neck) will usually involve muscle paralysis in all four limbs, generally called *quadriplegia. Paraplegia* involves muscle paralysis in the lower limbs and usually involves an injury to the spinal cord below the neck.

A spinal cord injury is usually responsive to rehabilitation, as persons with this injury generally do not encounter multiple handicaps. Physical activity provides an important positive outlet as well as a unique competitive challenge for students with spinal cord injuries. Many opportunities exist for successful mainstreaming of students with spinal cord injuries in physical activity or competitive athletics.

Instructional Adaptations for Paraplegics

- Require the student to perform all parts of the skill that he or she can do and provide a partner to perform other parts of the activity.
- Pair students whose skills complement each other.
- Preteach the skills with necessary adaptations such as using scooters or wheelchairs during a running activity.
- Try out the activities with the student prior to class to obtain a baseline of the student's ability.
- In activities that use the upper body, encourage the student to complete acquisition of the skill with maximum distance and accuracy. Concentrate on building the student's upper-body strength, flexibility, and endurance.
- If necessary, change the requirements of distance, accuracy, and/or form, but increase the number of repetitions.
- Emphasize exercises that increase circulation to lower limbs.

Environmental Adaptations for Paraplegics

- Use scooters, desk chairs with wheels, or athletic wheelchairs during locomotor activities.
- Teach the use of braces, parallel bars, crutches, and wheelchairs during locomotor activities.
- Attach elastic or string to objects to simplify their retrieval.

- Have the student transfer from the wheelchair to a mat during individualized activity to increase circulation to the lower limbs.
- Teach skills and activities in a swimming pool to counteract the effects of gravity.

Instructional Adaptations for Quadriplegics

- Substitute skills which need practice for those that are inappropriate; for example, practice breathing instead of jumping.
- Change the rules of the activity, so that if the student's chair moves an appropriate amount, a score is recorded for her or his team.
- Require the student to perform one part of a skill and ask a partner to perform other parts of the skill.
- Help the student to develop strength and endurance in the body parts that are capable of movement.
- Help the student become a knowledgeable spectator by demonstrating strategies for the activity on a board version.
- Encourage the student to give verbal directions to another student who can follow the directions and complete the movements.

Environmental Adaptations for Quadriplegics

- Consult an industrial arts department in the school district to help in designing and attaching paddles, shields, plows, and other aids and assistive devices to the student's wheelchair to facilitate involvement in activities.
- Use electric wheelchairs to allow the student greater independent mobility.
- Use a combination of attachments and electric controls to the wheelchair to allow the student to move into correct positions and intercept objects.
- Use foam balls and lightweight equipment.
- Provide a partner to push the student's wheelchair while the student in the wheelchair gives directions to the partner about where to go and at what speed.
- Use splints or assistive devices as suggested by an occupational or physical therapist.

Visual Impairments

Visual impairment is defined as a limitation in vision that, even with correction, adversely affects a student's educational performance. Vision impairment is classified into several categories. A *blind* student has substantial loss of sight for functional use. *Legally blind* students have visual acuity of 20/200 or less in the better eye with corrective lenses or a visual field of less than a 20-degree angle. *Partially sighted* students have a visual acuity between 20/70 and 20/200 with correction.

Often teachers and the visually impaired students are overly cautious and reluctant about participation in physical activities. The teacher must take an active role in preplanning and individual counseling to relieve students' fears about participating. Students with visual impairments tend to be stiff and often awkward in their movements; therefore, creative movements or relaxation techniques used as warm-up activities may be beneficial.

Emphasis in physical activities should be on individual improvement, optimizing the opportunity for the student to learn and experience motor skills for participation in lifetime physical activities.

Instructional Adaptations

- Allow the student to explore each day's arrangements for physical activities (set up) before the activity. Provide a sighted guide who will aid in familiarizing the student with the setting.
- Teach all students to use auditory and tactile cues in order to communicate with visually handicapped students during physical activities.
- Preteach rules so that the student can memorize this information. Call out directions during the activity.
- Allow the student to act out his or her role in the activity before adding other players.

Environmental Adaptations

- Use jointed dolls for models so that the student can simulate the motor skill steps of the activity with the doll.
- String guide ropes with knots to indicate distances to move in activities.
- Use noisemakers such as bells, cans, and whistles to indicate success, direction of targets and goals, or to alert the student to mistakes or obstacles.
- Give the student practice listening to the various sounds that different objects make in various locations; for example, demonstrate the sound of a ball bouncing off surfaces.
- Keep arrangements in the activity area consistent from one class session to the next.

Adapting the *Body Skills* Activities

With consideration of the characteristics of students with handicaps, a variety of adaptations can be made in the *Body Skills* activities.

Adapting Performance Objectives

The performance objectives may not accommodate the unique needs of some students. Following is a list of suggestions for adapting the performance objectives of the activities.

- If the student is unable to perform leg movements, he or she can perform creative arm movements.
- Allow the student to perform locomotor skills while sitting in a chair with wheels, or on a scooter.
- Allow partial participation by determining which parts of the skill or activity the student can perform.
- Substitute skills the student can adequately perform for those skills that the student cannot perform.
- Provide a partner to perform actions that the student is unable to perform.
- Emphasize accuracy in performance, rather than distance.
- Allow each student to perform the skill at his or her level of development for practice.
- Incorporate recommendations from physicians or therapists when planning the student's program.

Instructional Adaptations

The most flexible aspects of an activity are the directions. There are many different ways to modify an activity. When adapting the directions, it is important to modify traditional rules to create ways for students with handicaps to enjoy the activity. For example, shorten the goal distance and have students walk five steps, then jump once, instead of jumping all the way to the goal. The students themselves are often the best source of creative suggestions and adaptations to activities. If approached sensitively, social integration can be enhanced by asking students to suggest modifications that will make it possible for students with handicaps to participate. Following are some general guidelines and suggestions for adapting directions of the *Body Skills* activities.

- To give students with handicaps an equal opportunity for success, require other students to move in a more difficult manner, such as backward or in a crab walk or crawl.
- Pair students with a helper, guide, or buddy who will assist him or her in following directions and in completing the activity. In order to complement one another, each partner may perform parts of the skill.
- Emphasize competing with oneself, not with others. Establish baseline performance levels through pretesting students on new skills or activities. Chart progress to show improvements in performance.
- Allow the student to play a position that requires maximum action in a small area. For example, a blind student who has learned to serve and place a volleyball could serve every round.
- Adjust the rules of the activity to allow the student additional time, a greater number of steps, a shorter distance, or more pushes in a wheelchair to perform the desired skill.
- Modify the rules of the activity so that it is beneficial to the group to use the skills of the student with handicaps; for example, anytime the student performs a certain skill, the team is awarded additional points. These strategies emphasize cooperative setting of goals for small groups and rewarding and recognizing performance on the basis of group or individual performance.
- Establish and enforce a few clear, short rules with meaningful, natural consequences for the student. For example, if the student drops the ball, she or he must go back to the starting line and start over.
- Provide a partner to push the student's wheelchair while the student in the wheelchair gives the partner directions about where to go and at what speed.
- Provide balance and support by holding the student around the waist or under the arms.
- Preteach skills prior to the activity.
- Face the student and maintain eye contact while giving directions and demonstrating aspects of the activity.
- Use short, clear statements throughout instruction.
- Present lessons in a consistent manner.
- Give specific positive feedback for skills performed correctly. Give praise when warranted.

- Repeat important concepts or rules with the student just prior to the activity.
- Teach the student how to recognize social cues, body language, and voice intonations as part of the activity.
- Have a highly skilled student demonstrate actions while you point out specific details of the movements.
- Break the skill into smaller steps and teach sequential progression of each step to facilitate success.
- Demonstrate appropriate ways of showing anger.
- Use warm-ups and stretching prior to and just after the activity.
- Teach proper breathing techniques during the activity.
- Teach and demonstrate to the student how to pace him or herself.

Environmental Adaptations

- Vary the distances required for the student, or required for the other students, to recognize a student's disabilities.
- Allow the student to lean against a wall, table, or bar for support or balance.
- Mark small, defined areas for movement; for example, string guide ropes along the boundaries or paths to provide direction and organization of space.
- Use brightly colored objects or markings for boundaries, lines, targets, and fixtures.
- Incorporate music to control the speed and pace of movements in the activity.
- Use mirrors to highlight students' movements in activities.
- Eliminate any unnecessary equipment and distractions.
- Use bells, whistles, or other sounds as cues for targets and directions in the activity.
- Give visual, verbal, and tactile cues when giving directions; for example, use flashcards, bells, or flashing lights.
- Use assistive devices, such as walkers, tricycles, scooters, crutches, canes, braces, parallel bars, office chairs with wheels, wagons, to aid mobility and increase participation.
- Use a ceiling rope or a spotting belt to provide support to students with disabilities during the activity.
- Extend student's reach with floor hockey sticks, rackets, paddles, and/or batons.
- Attach elastic or string to objects to simplify their retrieval.
- Use brightly colored equipment.
- Provide adaptations to wheelchairs, such as shields or plows.
- Use sponge balls or yarn balls and other soft equipment.
- Use velcro straps to strap equipment, such as a bat, to the student to facilitate movements as well as for the safety of others.
- Use gripper gloves to help the student grasp an object.
- Attach ankle or wrist weights to relax the student's muscles.
- Attach bells or other devices to equipment for students who are visually impaired.

Appendix C

Body Skills *Materials*

The complete *Body Skills* program is contained in a portable carrying box that includes:

1 *Body Skills* Manual

1 Motor Skills Inventory (MSI) Record Booklet

1 Management Folder

31 Skill Folders
- 5 Body Management skills (green)
- 8 Locomotor skills (blue)
- 7 Body Fitness skills (red)
- 7 Object Movement skills (purple)
- 4 Fine Motor skills (orange)

103 Activity Cards, printed back to back

Body Management Activities

Body-Space Awareness
1. Fit as a Fiddle
2. Twister
3. Parachute Play
4. Scarf Fun
5. Who's the Leader?

Moving Balance
1. Connections
2. Safari
3. Beanbag Tag
4. Walk the Line
5. Canyon Cross
6. Copy Cats

Stationary Balance
1. Body Balances
2. Freeze!
3. Stay on the Rug
4. Number Balance
5. Team Balance
6. Circle Balance

Body Roll
1. Rock 'n Roll
2. Roll to the Gold
3. Tumbleweeds
4. People Bowling
5. Team Roll
6. Follow and Roll

Agility
1. Face to Face
2. Tiger Run
3. Left, Right, Full Speed Ahead
4. Hoops or Cones
5. Rock, Paper, or Scissors
6. Gold Rush

Locomotor Activities

Crawl
1. Carton Push
2. Animal Farm
3. Musical Crawl
4. Lion Tag
5. Troll Tag
6. Animal Trap

Walk
1. Tick Tock Walk
2. Eagles and Robins
3. Walk on Colors
4. Turtles and Bunnies
5. Bulls in a China Shop
6. Maze Craze

Horizontal Jump
1. Creature from Mars
2. Jump and Fetch
3. Mouse Catcher
4. Snake Charmer
5. Jump the Ditch
6. Crossing the River
7. Jump, Rabbit, Jump
8. Jungle Jumpers

Vertical Jump
1. Island Jumping
2. Johnny Jump Up
3. Green Tag
4. Jump the Rope
5. Reach for the Stars
6. Bowling for People

Run
1. Squirrels in Trees
2. Dogcatcher
3. Ghosts and Goblins
4. Fire Chief
5. Space Runners
6. Race and Chase
7. Carry Home the Bacon
8. Red Light, Green Light

Hop
1. Bunny Trap
2. Bee Sting
3. Double-Circle Hop
4. Walk-Hop Race
5. Carrot Grab
6. Bunny Tag
7. Hop to It
8. Bees in the Trees

Gallop
1. Gallop-Go-Round
2. Horse Pairs
3. Wild and Tame Horses
4. Gallop Away
5. O.K. Corral
6. Caravans

Skip
1. Circle Skip
2. Duck, Duck, Goose
3. Charlie Over the Water
4. Back 'n Forth
5. Scat
6. Cross the Meadow

Body Fitness Activities

Arm-Shoulder Flexibility
1. Twist and Turn
2. Book Pass
3. Tangle Town
4. Magic Wands
5. Sky Writing

Midbody Flexibility
1. Duck the Stick
2. Side to Side
3. Hoopla
4. Building Bridges
5. Wall Walk
6. Sweep

Aerobic Development
1. Huff 'n Puff Tag
2. Cross the USA
3. Color Hunt
4. Which Way?
5. Circle Tag
6. Jump Around the World

Abdominal Strength
1. Chin to Knees
2. Row the Boat
3. Spelling Bee
4. Ball Pass
5. Volley Balloon
6. Foot Catch

Leg-Hip Flexibility
1. Guard Your Goal
2. Stick Stack
3. Hold It
4. Inchworm Up
5. Mountain Climb
6. Stretch Tag

Leg-Hip Strength
1. Leg Wrestle
2. Stand Up
3. Stand Up, Sit Down, Jump, Jump, Jump
4. Inner Circle
5. Snake Pit
6. Partner Press

Arm-Shoulder Strength
1. Quicksand!
2. Blast Off
3. Work Your Way Around
4. Push or Pull
5. Survival
6. Monkeys and Apes

Object Movement Activities

Kick
1. Kick Off
2. Call and Kick
3. Through the Mountains
4. Circle Kick
5. Kick and Trade
6. Line Kick
7. Kick It Over
8. Guard Ball

Bounce
1. Number Bounce
2. The Coach Says
3. Odd 'n Even
4. Monster on the Loose
5. Circle Switch
6. Bounce It This Way
7. Go Ball
8. Dribble Baseball

Catch
1. Crystal Ball
2. Leader Ball
3. Pace Off
4. Inner Circle
5. Moon Shot
6. Cross Over
7. Monkeys in the Middle
8. Wall Ball
9. Big and Little

Overhand Throw
1. Step Back
2. Annie, Annie, Up and Over
3. Beanbag Toss
4. Sludge Ball
5. Run for Safety
6. Grizzly Toss
7. Beanbag Golf
8. Team Throw
9. Over the Net

Strike
1. Three Tees
2. Four Hits
3. Around the Order
4. Rebound Ball
5. Crowd Ball

Underhand Throw
1. Go for Ten
2. Box Ball
3. Hoop Bounce
4. Beanbag Horseshoe
5. Hoop Toss
6. Circle Toss

Underhand Roll
1. Knock the Box
2. Roll Away
3. Alley Ball
4. Team Ball
5. Roll Through
6. Rolling to the Green

Fine Motor Activities

Small-Object Control
1. Pass and Run
2. Pick Up
3. Bucket Brigade
4. Building Bigger Towers
5. Pinching Pennies
6. Pick Up Sticks

Grasp
1. Star Search
2. Reach, Reach
3. Pile Up
4. Ribbon Tag
5. Guess the Shape
6. There's a Hole in the Bucket
7. Making Mosaics
8. Drop the Bean

Hand Strength
1. Crumple and Toss
2. Howdy Partner
3. Wring Out the Sponge
4. Who's Got the Ball?
5. Newspaper Toss
6. Partner Tug-of-War

Visual-Motor Control
1. Tip-Top Tracing
2. Trace 'n Trade
3. Copycat
4. Beginning Writing
5. Chalkboard Copycat
6. Fancy Letters

35 Blackline Masters

- 1 Individual Skill Checklist
- 5 Class Record Forms
- 1 Individual Educational Planning Form
- 28 Activity Sheets for use with Visual-Motor Control Activities

Appendix D
Sample Yearly Program Plan Using the Body Skills *Curriculum*

september

sunday	monday	tuesday	wednesday	thursday	friday	saturday
		1	2	3	4	5
6	7	8	9 MSI Assessment	10	11 MSI assessment	12
13	14 MSI Assessment	15	16 Aerobic Dev 1* Run 1 Underhand Roll 1	17	18 Aerobic Dev 2 Run 2 Underhand Roll 2	19
20	21 Aerobic Dev 1 (Variation) Run 3 Underhand Roll 2 (Var)	22	23 Aerobic Dev 2 (Var) Run 4 Underhand Roll 3	24	25 Aerobic Dev 2 (Var) Run 1 (Var) Underhand Roll 3 (Var)	26
27	28 Arm Flex 1 Run 2 (Var) Kick 1	29	30 Arm Flex 1 (Var) Run 3 (Var) Kick 2			

october

sunday	monday	tuesday	wednesday	thursday	friday	saturday
				1	2 Arm-Sh Flex 2 Run 4 (Var) Kick 1 (Var)	3
4	5 Arm-Sh Flex 2 (Var) H Jump 1 Kick 2 (Var)	6	7 Arm-Sh Flex 3 H Jump 1 (Var) Kick 3	8	9 Aerobic Dev 5 H Jump 2 Kick 3 (Var)	10
11	12 Aerobic Dev 6 H Jump 3 Kick 4	13	14 Catch 1 H Jump 4 Kick 4 (Var)	15	16 Catch 2 H Jump 4 (Var) Kick 5	17
18	19 Catch 3 H Jump 5 Kick 5 (Var)	20	21 Catch 4 Leg-Hip Strength 1 Kick 6	22 Conferences	23	24
25	26 Catch 5 Leg-Hip Strength 2 Kick 6 (Var)	27	28 Catch 6 Leg-Hip Strength 3 Hop 1	29	30 Halloween Choice Day	31

*Activity number

november

sunday	monday	tuesday	wednesday	thursday	friday	saturday
1	2 Body Roll 3 Midbody Flex 4 Hop 2	3	4 Body Roll 3 (Var) Bounce 1 Hop 1 (Var)	5	6 Body Roll 4 Bounce 2 Hop 2 (Var)	7
8	9 Bounce 2 (Var) Run 3 Hop 3	10	11 Bounce 3 Run 3 (Var) Hop 3 (Var)	12	13 School Assembly — No Class	14
15	16 Bounce 4 Run 4 Hop 3 (Var)	17	18 Bounce 3 (Var) Run 4 (Var) Hop 4	19	20 Bounce 4 (Var) Run 2 (Var) Hop 4 (Var)	21
22	23 School Assembly No Class	24	25 Agility 1 Arm-Sh Flex 3 (Var) Gallop 1	26 Thanksgiving Holiday	27	28
29	30 Agility 2 Arm-Sh Flex 4 Gallop 2					

december

sunday	monday	tuesday	wednesday	thursday	friday	saturday
		1	2 Agility 2 (Var) Arm-Sh Flex 4 (Var) Gallop 1 (Var)	3	4 Agility 3 Arm-Sh Flex 5 Gallop 2 (Var)	5
6	7 Agility 4 Arm-Sh Flex 5 (Var) Gallop 3	8	9 Gallop 3 (Var) S Balance 1 Leg-Hip Flex 1	10	11 Gallop 4 S Balance 1 (Var) Leg-Hip Flex 1 (Var)	12
13	14 Gallop 4 (Var) S Balance 2 Leg-Hip Flex 2	15	16 Gallop 5 S Balance 2 (Var) Leg-Hip Flex 2 (Var)	17	18 Gallop 5 (Var) S Balance 3 Leg-Hip Flex 2 (Var)	19
20	21 Gallop 6 S Balance 3 (Var) Agility 1 (Var)	22	23 Holiday ———	24 ———	25 ———	26
27	28 Holiday ———	29 ———	30 ———	31 ———		

january

sunday	monday	tuesday	wednesday	thursday	friday	saturday
					1	2
3	4 Gallop 6 (Var) S Balance 3 (Var) Agility 2 (Var)	5	6 Gallop 6 (Var) S Balance 4 Agility 3 (Var)	7	8 Aerobic Dev 2 V Jump 1 Catch 1	9
10	11 Aerobic Dev 2 (Var) V Jump 1 (Var) Catch 1 (Var)	12	13 Aerobic Dev 3 V Jump 1 (Var) Catch 2	14	15 Aerobic Dev 3 (Var) V Jump 2 O Throw 1	16
17	18 Abdominal Strength 2 O Throw 2 M Balance 2 (Var)	19	20 Abdominal Strength 2 (Var) O Throw 2 (Var) M Balance 3	21	22 Abdominal Strength 2 (Var) O Throw 3 M Balance 3 (Var)	23
24 31	25 Midbody Flex 2 O Throw 3 (Var) Body Roll 1	26	27 Midbody Flex 2 (Var) O Throw 3 (Var) Body Roll 2	28	29 Midbody Flex 3 O Throw 3 (Var) Body Roll 2 (Var)	30

february

sunday	monday	tuesday	wednesday	thursday	friday	saturday
	1 Midbody Flex 1 Bounce 3 Body Roll 3	2	3 Midbody Flex 1 (Var) Bounce 3 (Var) Body Roll 3 (Var)	4	5 Midbody Flex 2 Bounce 4 Body Roll 4	6
7	8 Aerobic Dev 1 Bounce 4 (Var) Body-Sp. Awareness 1 (Var)	9	10 Abdominal Strength 2 Bounce 5 Body-Sp. Awareness 2	11	12 Abdominal Strength 2 (Var) Bounce 5 (Var) Body Sp Awareness 2 (Var)	13
14	15 Abdominal Strength 3 Catch 2 Body-Sp Awareness 3	16	17 Aerobic Dev 1 (Var) Catch 2 (Var) Body-Sp. Awareness 3 (Var)	18	19 Arm-Sh. Strength 2 Catch 3 Agility 2	20
21	22 Arm-Sh. Strength 2 (Var) Catch 3 (Var) Agility 2 (Var)	23	24 Arm-Sh. Strength 3 Catch 4 Agility 3	25	26 Choice Day	27
28	29 Leg-Hip Strength 2 Skip 1 M Balance 2					

march

sunday	monday	tuesday	wednesday	thursday	friday	saturday
		1	2 Leg-Hip Strength 3 Skip 2 M Balance 3	3	4 Leg-Hip Strength 3 (Var.) Skip 3 M Balance 3 (Var.)	5
6	7 Leg-Hip Strength 3 (Var.) Skip 4 U Throw 1	8	9 Leg-Hip Strength 4 Skip 4 (Var.) U. Throw 2	10	11 Aerobic Dev 2 Skip 5 U Throw 3	12
13	14 Leg-Hip Flex 1 Run 5 U Throw 3 (Var.)	15	16 Leg-Hip Flex 1 (Var.) Run 5 (Var.) U Throw 4	17	18 Conferences	19
20	21 Abdominal Strength 3 Run 6 Catch 2 (Var.)	22	23 Abdominal Strength 3 (Var.) Run 6 (Var.) Catch 3 (Var.)	24	25 Abdominal Strength 4 H. Jump 5 (Var.) Catch 4 (Var.)	26
27	28 Aerobic Dev 2 (Var.) H. Jump 6 Catch 5 (Var.)	29	30 Aerobic Dev 3 H Jump 6 (Var.) Catch 6	31		

april

sunday	monday	tuesday	wednesday	thursday	friday	saturday
					1 No school	2
3	4 Holiday	5	6	7	8	9
10	11 Aerobic Dev 3 (Var.) Hop 3 Strike 1	12	13 Aerobic Dev 3 (Var.) Hop 3 (Var.) Strike 1 (Var.)	14	15 Aerobic Dev 4 Hop 4 Strike 2	16
17	18 Midbody Flex 2 Skip 2 Strike 2 (Var.)	19	20 Midbody Flex 2 (Var.) Skip 2 (Var.) Strike 3	21	22 Midbody Flex 3 Skip 2 (Var.) Strike 3 (Var.)	23
24	25 Midbody Flex 3 (Var.) Skip 3 Strike 4	26	27 Aerobic Dev. 4 (Var.) Gallop 2 Body Roll 2	28	29 Aerobic Dev 5 Gallop 2 Body Roll 2 (Var.)	30

may

sunday	monday	tuesday	wednesday	thursday	friday	saturday
1	2 Aerobic Dev 1 Run 3 O Throw 2	3	4 Aerobic Dev 1 (Var) Run 3 (Var) O Throw 2 (Var)	5	6 Aerobic Dev 2 Run 3 (Var) O Throw 3	7
8	9 Arm-Sh. Strength 2 (Var) Run 4 O Throw 3 (Var)	10	11 Arm-Sh. Strength 3 Run 4 (Var) O Throw 4	12	13 Arm-Sh. Strength 3 (Var) Run 4 (Var) O Throw 4 (Var)	14
15	16 Arm-Sh. Flex 2 H. Jump 2 Strike 3	17	18 Arm-Sh. Flex 2 (Var) H. Jump 2 (Var) Strike 3 (Var)	19	20 Arm-Sh. Flex 3 H. Jump 3 Strike 4	21
22	23 Aerobic Dev 3 (Var) H. Jump 3 (Var) Strike 4 (Var)	24	25 Aerobic Dev 4 (Var) H. Jump 4 Strike 5	26	27 Aerobic Dev 5 H. Jump 4 (Var) Strike 5 (Var)	28
29	30 Holiday	31				

june

sunday	monday	tuesday	wednesday	thursday	friday	saturday
			1 MSI Assessment	2	3 MSI Assessment	4
5	6 MSI assessment	7	8	9	10	11
12	13	14	15	16	17	18
19	20	21	22	23	24	25
26	27	28	29	30		

Appendix E

Field Testers

The following people participated in the second field test in the spring of 1985.

Linda Ansell
Fifth Grade Teacher
Palo Verde Elementary School
Palo Verde, California

Russell Bakko
Adaptive Physical Education Coordinator
Mounds View Public Schools
Roseville, Minnesota

Vicky Blank
Adaptive Physical Education Specialist
Bonita Unified School District
San Dimas, California
Claremont Unified School District
Claremont, California

Kim Bloom
Adaptive Physical Education Teacher
Madison Elementary School
Blaine, Minnesota

Madelene Canine
Kindergarten Teacher
El Carmelo Elementary School
Palo Alto, California

Dan Cariaga
Adaptive Physical Education Specialist
Hacienda La Puente Unified School District
La Puente, California

Alice Ann Chandler
Second-Third Grade Teacher
El Carmelo Elementary School
Palo Alto, California

Gail Crotty
Adaptive Physical Education Specialist
Alhambra School District
Alhambra, California
South Pasadena Unified School District
South Pasadena, California

Ruth Donnelly
Second Grade Teacher
El Carmelo Elementary School
Palo Alto, California

Melanie Easley
Physical Education Teacher
Watson Elementary School
Garland, Texas

Leilani Eng
Third-Fourth Grade Teacher
El Carmelo Elementary School
Palo Alto, California

Dorothy England
Adaptive Physical Education Specialist
Hacienda La Puente Unified School District
La Puente, California

Norman Feig
Physical Education Specialist
Northgate Elementary School
Bloomington, Minnesota

Delores Froehlich
Special Day Class Teacher
San Gabriel Elementary School District
San Gabriel, California

Jean Gong
First Grade Teacher
El Carmelo Elementary School
Palo Alto, California

Georgia Hall
Adaptive Physical Education Specialist
Paramount Unified School District
Paramount, California

Dean Hamre
Elementary Physical Education Consultant
Washington Elementary School
Anoka, Minnesota

Elizabeth Harris
Physical Education Teacher
Sally B. Elliot Elementary School
Irving, Texas

Ken Hill
Adaptive Physical Education Specialist
San Jose Unified School District
San Jose, California

Lydia Hood
Physical Education Teacher
John Townley Elementary School
Irving, Texas

Marianne Johnsen
Fourth-Fifth Grade Teacher
El Carmelo Elementary School
Palo Alto, California

Diana Junger
Physical Education Teacher
Garland Independent Schools
Garland, Texas

Judy Jungwirth
Physical Education Specialist
Poplar Bridge Elementary School
Bloomington, Minnesota

Juli Kennedy
Adaptive Physical Education Specialist
Monrovia Unified School District
Monrovia, California

Beverly Kerby
Physical Education Teacher
Park Crest Elementary School
Garland, Texas

Lisa Kerwien-Harman
Second Grade Teacher
Palo Verde Elementary School
Palo Alto, California

Steve Knop
Adaptive Physical Education Teacher
Sordeberg Elementary School
Coon Rapids, Minnesota

Mitch Lewis
Adaptive Physical Education Specialist
San Jose Unified School District
San Jose, California

Dan McEachran
Physical Education Teacher
Susan Lindgren Elementary School
St. Louis Park, Minnesota

Jerry Miller
Physical Education Teacher
Valentine Hills Elementary School
Mounds View, Minnesota

Eileen Nelson
Physical Education Teacher
Hillcrest Elementary School
Bloomington, Minnesota

Nora Pederson
Adaptive Physical Education Specialist
Downey Unified School District
Downey, California

Kathy Preston
Adaptive Physical Education Specialist
San Marino Unified School District
San Marino, California

Beverly Purdom
Physical Education Teacher
Montclair Elementary School
Garland, Texas

Clyde Riddel
Adaptive Physical Education Specialist
Robert Louis Stevenson Elementary School
Fridley, Minnesota

Diane Savitt
Adaptive Physical Education Teacher
St. Louis Park Public Schools
St. Louis Park, Minnesota

Michael Schneider
Physical Education Teacher
Caldwell Elementary School
Garland, Texas

Laura Schutman
Special Day Class Teacher
San Gabriel Elementary School
District
San Gabriel, California

Susan Shamburger
Physical Education Teacher
John Haley Elementary School
Irving, Texas

Lynn Sieving
Physical Education Teacher
Peter Hobart Elementary School
St. Louis Park, Minnesota

Marsha Vawter
Physical Education Teacher
Lee Britain Elementary School
Irving, Texas

Joanie Verderber
Adaptive Physical Education
Specialist
San Gabriel Elementary School
District
San Gabriel, California

Sue Wheeler-Ayres
Adaptive Physical Education
Specialist
San Jose Unified School District
San Jose, California

Jack Willhite
Adaptive Physical Education Teacher
St. Louis Park Public Schools
St. Louis Park, Minnesota

Joan Winsor
Special Education Teacher
El Carmelo Elementary School
Palo Alto, California

Annie Yount
Fifth-Sixth Grade Teacher
El Carmelo Elementary School
Palo Alto, California

Glossary

balance beam—six- to ten-foot wooden beam that may vary in width from two to six inches and sits two-inches to four feet above the floor; often used for balance activities

body image, body cognition—awareness of one's own body demonstrated by identifying self in a photograph or mirror and identifying one's body parts; knowing the capabilities and limitations of body movements

cargo net—ropes knotted in a squared pattern to look like a large net and hung from the ceiling or wall for students to climb

carpet square—carpet sample no less than one foot square

ceiling ropes—large ropes knotted at the ends and hung from a gymnasium ceiling for students to climb

coordination—the ability to move one's body in a smooth, integrated manner; for example, moving the arms and legs simultaneously and smoothly while doing jumping jacks

copy—copy a stimulus drawing in an adjacent space or from a distance

cues—a signal, word, or phrase given to students to begin a specific action. Instructional cues can be auditory (words, whistles), visual (pictures, flashcards, demonstration), or tactile (touching and physically guiding student movements).

directionality—skill in moving in different directions in space (right, left, forward, backward, up, down)

dominant hand—hand that is most effective, preferred, or predominant in movement

equilibrium—a state of stationary or moving balance

extension—straightening and stretching a limb to result in increasing the angle between the bones of a limb at the joint

figure-ground perception—the ability to recognize an object in the foreground as separate in space from objects in the background; in catching, to be able to see the ball clearly from the time it is thrown until it is caught

flat-footed—steps characteristic of an immature walk or gallop, in which the heel and toe strike the floor simultaneously, making a slapping sound

flexibility—the ability to move a joint through its full range of motion; to easily flex and extend muscles to their maximum range

follow through—continuing a throwing or kicking motion after contact with the ball or other object; in throwing, continuing to move the hand and arm in the direction of the receiver or target; in kicking, continuing to move the foot and leg in the direction the ball was kicked

foot dribbling—moving a ball forward using little kicks made with the inside of the foot, alternating feet

functional—middle level of skill performance in which the basic movements are performed adequately but slightly awkwardly

heel-toe—steps in which the toe of the back foot touches the heel of the front foot *heel-to-toe strike/pattern*—steps in which the heel touches the floor first and then the foot rolls forward and down so the toe is touching the floor as the heel is lifted and the foot comes up off the floor

laterality—the ability to move to the right or left as desired or directed

mature—highest level of skill performance, in which the movements are performed in a smooth, integrated manner

monkey bars/jungle gym—playground equipment usually made from connected bars on which children climb or swing from their arms

opposition—moving body parts in opposite directions; in walking, a movement pattern in which the right arm swings forward as the left leg steps forward, and the left arm and right knee are back

overhand—action in which the hand moves forward and down from above shoulder level

palmer grasp—taking hold of an object by wrapping fingers and thumb around it, enveloping the object in the palm of the hand

parachute—large, umbrella-shaped device made from lightweight fabric used in movement activities; defective airplane parachutes may be used

pincer grasp—picking up a small object with the thumb and forefinger while the other fingers are curled toward the palm

points of support—parts of the body touching the floor; for example, the feet provide two points of support when a person is standing

range of motion—movement of a joint from its minimum through its maximum angle

reflex—automatic, unconscious, and often inborn response to a stimulus

resistance—exerting force in opposition to a movement, as exercising with weights adds resistance to muscles and increases strength

rudimentary—lowest level of skill performance, in which the basic movements are performed but in an awkward, uncoordinated manner

scooter—close-to-the-floor square or rectangular platform on four wheels on which students can sit, kneel, or lie as they move themselves with their hands or legs

signal—a signal or sound used consistently to indicate the beginning of an activity. The signal should include a visual element, such as a raised flag, for hearing-impaired students.

spotter—a person who stands beside a person who is performing a physical stunt to provide support. A spotter may put one or both hands on the performing student's waist, or hold hands near the student to provide support as needed.

straddle—to sit, stand, or walk with legs wide apart

task specific—pertaining to a particular task or action

trace—draw directly over lines or a design as accurately as possible

underhand—action in which the hand moves forward and up from below shoulder level

vaulting box/block—an apparatus, usually made from wood, that is supported in a horizontal position above the floor, used in vaulting or gymnastic exercises

weight transfer—shifting one's body weight from one foot or side of the body to the other; for example, stepping forward while throwing

References

Bagley, N.A. 1935. "The Development of Motor Abilities During the First Three Years." Society of Research in Child Development 1:1-26.

Brackbill, Y., ed. 1967. *Infancy and Early Childhood.* New York: Free Press.

Bruininks, R.H. 1974. "Physical and Motor Development of Retarded Persons." In *International Review of Research in Mental Retardation.* Vol. 7, edited by N.R. Ellis. New York: Academic Press.

———. 1978. *Bruininks-Oseretsky Test of Motor Proficiency.* Circle Pines, MN: American Guidance Service.

Bruininks, R.H., R.W. Woodcock, R.F. Weatherman, and B.K. Hill. 1985. *Scales of Independent Behavior.* Allen, TX: DLM/Teaching Resources.

Corbin, C.B. 1973. *A Textbook of Motor Development.* Dubuque, IA: Wm. C. Brown.

Cratty, B.J. 1972. *Physical Expressions of Intelligence.* Englewood Cliffs, NJ: Prentice Hall.

———. 1979. *Perceptual and Motor Development in Infants and Children.* Englewood Cliffs, NJ: Prentice-Hall.

Cronbach, L.J. 1963. "Course Improvement Through Evaluation." *Teachers College Record* 64:672-683.

Espenschade, A.S., and H.M. Eckert. 1967. *Motor Development.* Columbus, OH: Merrill.

———. 1980. *Motor Development.* 2d ed. Columbus, OH: Merrill.

Fleishman, E.A. 1964. *The Structure and Measurement of Physical Fitness.* Englewood Cliffs, NJ: Prentice-Hall.

Gallahue, D.L. 1976. *Motor Development and Movement Experiences for Young Children.* New York: Wiley.

Gerhardt, L.A. 1973. *Moving and Knowing.* Englewood Cliffs, NJ: Prentice-Hall.

Gesell, A.L. 1940. *The First Five Years of a Child's Life.* New York: Harper and Row.

Grossman, H.S., ed. 1983. *Manual on Terminology and Classification in Mental Retardation.* Washington, D.C.: American Association on Mental Deficiency.

Guilford, J.P. 1958. "A System of Psychomotor Abilities." *American Journal of Psychology* 71:164-174.

Guttridge, M.V. 1939. "A Study of Motor Achievements of Young Children." *Arch.Psychol.* 244:1.

Halvorson, L.E., and M.A. Robertson. 1966. "A Study of Motor Pattern Development in Young Children." Report to the National Convention of the American Association of Health, Physical Education, and Recreation (AAHPER), Chicago.

Hambleton, R.K., and L.L. Cook. 1977. "Latent Trait Models and Their Use in the Analysis of Educational Test Data." *Journal of Educational Measurement* 14:75-96.

Harrow, A.J. 1972. *Taxonomy of the Psychomotor Domain: A Guide for Developing Behavior Objectives.* New York: David McKay.

Ilg, F.L., and L.B. Ames. 1966. *School Readiness.* New York: Harper and Row.

Jenkins, L.M. 1930. *A Comparative Study of Motor Achievements of Children Five, Six, and Seven Years of Age.* New York: Teacher's College, Columbia University.

Koegh, J. 1965. *Motor Performance of Elementary School Children.* Department of Physical Education, University of California, Los Angeles.

Lord, F.M. 1980. *Application of Item Response Theory to Practical Testing Problems.* Hillsdale, NJ: Eribaum.

———. 1960. "Large-Sample Covariance Analysis When the Central Variable is Fallible." *Journal of the American Statistical Association.* 55:307-321.

Poe, A. 1976. "Description of the Movement Characteristics of Two-Year-Old Children Performing the Jump and Reach." *Research Quarterly, American Association of Health and Physical Education* 47:260.

Public Law 94-142. 1975. Education for All Handicapped Children Act of 1975. 94th Congress, S.6 (20 USC 1401), November 29, 1975.

Rarick, G.L. 1961. *Motor Development During Infancy and Childhood.* Madison, WI: College Printing and Typing Co.

Rarick, G.L., and D.A. Dobbins. 1972. *Basic Components in the Motor Performance of EMR Children: Implications for Curriculum Development.* (Grant No. OEG-0-70-2568-610). Washington, D.C.: U.S. Office of Education.

Rasch, G. 1960. *Probablistic Models for Some Intelligence and Attainment Tests.* Copenhagen: Danish Institute for Educational Research.

Richman, N., J. Stevenson, and P.J. Graham. 1982. *Preschool to School: A Behavioral Study.* New York: Academic Press.

Sinclair, C.B. 1973. *Movement of the Young Child.* Columbus, OH: Merrill.

Stake, R.E. 1967. "Toward a Technology for the Evaluation of Educational Programs." In *Perspectives of Curriculum Evaluation,* edited by R.W. Tyler, R.M. Gagne, and M. Scriven. AERA Monograph Series on Curriculum Evaluation. Chicago: Rand McNally.

Von Bertalanffy, L. 1968. *General System Theory.* New York: George Braziller.

Wellman, B. 1937. "Motor Achievements of Preschool Children." *Childhood Education* 13:311.

Wickstrom, R.L. 1977. *Fundamental Motor Patterns.* Philadelphia: Lea and Febiger.

Woodcock, R.W. 1978. *Development and Standardization of the Woodcock-Johnson Psycho-Educational Battery.* Allen, TX: DLM/Teaching Resources.

Wright, B.D. 1968. Sample-Free Test Calibration and Person Measurement. Proceedings of the 1967 Invitational Conference on Testing Problems. Princeton NJ: Educational Testing Service.

Wright, B.D., and B.H. Stone. 1979. *Best Test Design.* Chicago: MESA Press.